4-
1/20

Terry Cascino
President AAN

With best wishes,

Raad Shakir
President WFN

Vancouver 2016

The History of the World
Federation of Neurology

The History of the World Federation of Neurology
The First 50 Years

Johan A. Aarli

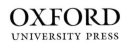

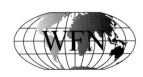

OXFORD
UNIVERSITY PRESS

Great Clarendon Street, Oxford, OX2 6DP,
United Kingdom

Oxford University Press is a department of the University of Oxford.
It furthers the University's objective of excellence in research, scholarship,
and education by publishing worldwide. Oxford is a registered trade mark of
Oxford University Press in the UK and in certain other countries

© Oxford University Press 2014

The moral rights of the author have been asserted

First Edition published in 2014

Impression: 1

All rights reserved. No part of this publication may be reproduced, stored in
a retrieval system, or transmitted, in any form or by any means, without the
prior permission in writing of Oxford University Press, or as expressly permitted
by law, by licence or under terms agreed with the appropriate reprographics
rights organization. Enquiries concerning reproduction outside the scope of the
above should be sent to the Rights Department, Oxford University Press, at the
address above

You must not circulate this work in any other form
and you must impose this same condition on any acquirer

Published in the United States of America by Oxford University Press
198 Madison Avenue, New York, NY 10016, United States of America

British Library Cataloguing in Publication Data
Data available

Library of Congress Control Number: 2014932763

ISBN 978–0–19–871306–7

Printed and bound by
CPI Group (UK) Ltd, Croydon, CR0 4YY

Whilst every effort has been made to ensure that the contents of this work
are as complete, accurate and-up-to-date as possible at the date of writing,
Oxford University Press is not able to give any guarantee or assurance that
such is the case. Readers are urged to take appropriately qualified medical
advice in all cases. The information in this work is intended to be useful to the
general reader, but should not be used as a means of self-diagnosis or for the
prescription of medication.

Links to third party websites are provided by Oxford in good faith and
for information only. Oxford disclaims any responsibility for the materials
contained in any third party website referenced in this work.

Foreword

Writing as I do in my 90th year, I can say truthfully and with a sense of pleasure and pride that the World Federation of Neurology has played an important part in my professional life. This book, skilfully and judiciously written by my good friend and colleague Professor Johan Aarli is without question a major scholarly work based upon careful historical research and an encyclopedic knowledge of the origins of the organization and of its development over the last 50 years. In the individual chapters he sketches the situation of world neurology before the organization was conceived, its establishment, first in embryo and then in infancy under the inspired leadership of Ludo van Bogaert, and then its subsequent development through adolescence and into maturity, concluding finally with cogent observations about the present standing of the organization, its relationship to professional societies, to regional neurological congresses, and to the World Health Organization, bearing in mind its increasingly vital role in influencing leadership, teaching, and research in the clinical neurosciences worldwide.

This fascinating story describes how, in its early months and years, the Federation was enabled to function and expand through funding from the US National Institutes of Health (NIH), which allowed the WFN to establish Problem Commissions dealing with individual areas in the clinical neurosciences. Regional developments in the Americas, in Europe, in the Middle East, and in Asia and Oceania were sponsored, leading ultimately to the development of pan-American, pan-European, pan-Arab, -African, -Asian and -Oceanian congresses, each affiliated to the WFN. The book describes sensitively but effectively the major problems which arose when the NIH money ran out, and the crucial Geneva meeting at which the Problem Commissions were disbanded and were replaced by a research committee closely integrated with the WFN and representing self-supporting research groups, many of which eventually matured into international societies. Professor Aarli also notes the inter-relationship between developments in neuroscience on the one hand and world affairs on the other, thus highlighting historical inter-relationships, and he does not avoid mentioning the strengths and possible weaknesses of some of those involved in the organization and development of the Federation. Plainly, when the WFN became responsible, in collaboration with its research committee, for the organization of world congresses of neurology, and was able to negotiate arrangements with the host societies which were of mutual financial benefit, the funding of the WFN became much more secure, a process which was enhanced when a permanent office was established and the organization became a registered charity and a company limited by guarantee. Clearly described throughout is the debt owed by the WFN, not only to its presidents, but also to secretaries, treasurers-general, and chairmen of committees, but also, in the more recent past, to its trustees. The crucial role played by the WFN in promoting the development of the clinical neurosciences in relatively undeveloped countries is made clear throughout, and we can now say with some pride that the influence of the Federation on neurology throughout the world has been sustained.

I am personally honoured and delighted to have played some small part in the organization throughout its, at times, uneven progress, and was immensely honoured by being awarded the WFN Medal at the 20th World Congress in Morocco in 2011. Posterity will be very grateful to Professor Aarli for this historical work of scholarship.

Lord Walton of Detchant   John Walton,
Northumberland   Kt TD MA MD DSc FRCP FMedSci

Preface

This is not a book on the history of neurology. It is an attempt to write the history of the World Federation of Neurology (WFN).

The clinical specialty of neurology developed in the second part of the 19th century. In many countries, neurological departments had been established more than 50 years before the WFN was founded in 1957. The history of the WFN has therefore little to do with the history of the development and progress in the neurosciences. It is much more integrated in the development of international collaboration in neurology, with dissemination of information, the need to learn from each other, independent of political systems. The WFN is an apolitical organization, but has a basis in the development of democracy worldwide.

There were international congresses in neurology (and other parts of medicine) in the 19th century. But 'the world' in a pre-1900 context meant 'the western world', and one national neurological association usually organized international conferences. A World Congress is sponsored by an international society, which assumes responsibility for the organization of the meeting. Such institutions first became established after the Second World War.

Johan A. Aarli

Acknowledgements

Many people helped me prepare this book on the history of the first 50 years of the World Federation of Neurology. First and foremost, I am thankful to Dr. Lewis P. Rowland for his chapter on Houston Merritt and Pearce Bailey, who were of critical importance in the shaping of the organization. My warmest personal thanks go to the group of neurologists with whom I have been working during and after my eight years of service to the WFN, as First Vice President (2002–2005), then as President (2006–2009). They include Jun Kimura, who was President, and Richard Godwin-Austen, Secretary-Treasurer General, during my first four years. And they include Marianne de Visser, William Carroll, Raad Shakir, Ryuji Kaji, Vladimir Hachinski, Werner Hacke, Roger Rosenberg, Gustavo Roman, and Theodore Munsat, who have been WFN officers during my administration. They have all been loyal, hard-working colleagues and are also personal friends.

I am deeply thankful to Mr Keith Newton, who has been the WFN Administrator as long as I have been associated with the WFN and who represents the institutional memory of the Federation. Ms Susan Bilger and Ms Laura Druce are secretaries at the WFN Secretariat and have been very helpful in my work. Professor James F. Toole was my mentor in establishing the contact with WHO. I am very grateful to him for our long-lasting collaboration and friendship. The Africa Initiative is a central part of my involvement with the WFN. Amadou Gallo Diop of Dakar (Senegal) and Alfred Njamnshi of Yaounde (Cameroon) are key persons who made the initiative a part of the WFN programme, and it was Gallo who first coined the term 'with Africa, for Africa'. Pierre Bill of Durban (South Africa), Michel Dumas of Limoges (France), Rajesh Kalaria of Newcastle (UK), and Girish Modi of Johannesburg (South Africa) have contributed effectively in linking Africa to the Global Neurological Community. I would also like to address warm words of thank to my colleagues who have been instrumental in preparing the neurology specialty training programmes for African neurologists in Rabat, Morocco, and Cairo, Egypt, Mohamed S. El-Tamawi of Cairo (Egypt), El Alaoui Faris of Rabat (Morocco), Ragnar Stien of Oslo (Norway). Ahmed Khalifa of Damascus (Syria) has written the chapter on the PAUNS, and Man Mohan Mendiratta the chapter on neurology in India. I have had the great pleasure of meeting and collaborating with colleagues who have been central in developing the regional neurological associations: the founder of the European Federation of Neurological Societies, Franz Gerstenbrand of Vienna (Austria), Riadh Gouider (Tunisia) and Ahmed Khalifa of Damascus (Syria), both representing the Pan Arab Region (PAUNS), Alfred Njamnshi of Cameroon of the Pan African Association of Neurological Sciences (PAANS), Amado San Luis on the Philippines, Man Mohan Mendiratta on neurology in India, for which I am very thankful.

Johan A. Aarli

Contents

1 Neurology before the World Federation of Neurology *1*

2 The Shaping of the Organization *11*

3 The World Federation of Neurology: Structure and Organization *85*

4 The World Federation of Neurology Applied Research Committee *109*

5 Communication in the World Federation of Neurology *139*

6 Regional Neurological Associations *147*

7 The World Federation of Neurology and the World Health Organization *167*

8 In Service of the World Federation of Neurology *173*

9 The International (World) Congresses of Neurology *187*

10 Epilogue *205*

Appendix 1: Memorandum and Articles of Association *211*

Index *227*

Chapter 1

Neurology before the World Federation of Neurology

Neurologists who met at international meetings in the early 1950s informally discussed the shaping of an international organization from the existing national neurological societies. They hoped that such a federation would contribute to the dissemination of information and to scientific progress in the neurosciences. At that time, the contact between research groups in various countries was weak and had been insufficient during the Cold War. International and especially intercontinental travelling was complicated and expensive. There was a hope that the existence of an international organization for neurology would create programmes of basic and clinical research in the neurosciences. Such an organization might also promote the development of neurological services in developing countries, many of them at that time still colonies of European powers. This contributed to the formation of the World Federation of Neurology (WFN).

The history of the WFN has three different aspects. The backbone—the history of the formation and expansion of the organization and its development during its presidencies is one part. Another element is the development of the WFN structure, with its committees and sub-organizations and the dramatic growth of the WFN Research Groups. They reflect neurology during the last 50 years. The third element is represented by the World Congresses of Neurology.

The WFN was founded during the Sixth World Congress of Neurosciences, which was held in Brussels in 1957. The first international congress of neurosciences in which WFN was involved took place in Rome in September 1961. The first six congresses have since been included in the sequence of World Congresses of Neurology, although they took place before the WFN was founded.

The World Congress of Medicine (London 1913)

In August 1913, 5546 active participants met in London for the 17th World Congress of Medicine. In his opening address, Sir Thomas Barlow, president of the Royal College of Physicians of London, reviewed the developments in medicine since the previous world congress, which had taken place 32 years earlier in London in 1881.

There had been international medical congresses previously: the first was in 1867 in Paris, the second in 1869 in Florence, the third in 1873 in Vienna, the fourth in 1875 in Brussels, the fifth in 1877 in Geneva, and the sixth in 1879 in Amsterdam.

What made the 1881 Congress different from the previous and from the following? First, it became the largest and most successful ever. At each international congress in medicine, new sciences in medicine had been presented, and the London Congress 1881 was a landmark in the general acceptance of the role of the new science of bacteriology.

At London in 1913, neurology found its place. There were specific sections for the various medical specialties. Fred Batten served as secretary for the section of neurology, and as the editor of the Congress Proceedings. Joseph Babinski, Auguste Tournay, and Max Rothmann discussed 'Cerebellar symptoms', Jules Dejerine 'Motor Aphasia, Anarthria, and Apraxia', and Hermann Oppenheim and William G. Spiller reviewed myopathy disorders. Neurosyphilis was an important topic, and Paul Ehrlich gave a plenary session on 'Chemo-Therapy'.

The Horsley–Clarke frame was demonstrated at the congress. It was extensively used throughout the next four decades for excitation and lesion production in experimental animals. Robert Henry Clarke and the pioneer neurosurgeon Victor Horsley had developed it in 1906 for making brain lesions.

Many participants at the world congress believed that the world was now entering a period of peace and stability. The American delegate, Alfred Reginald Allen, concluded in his farewell speech at the end of the congress:

> And now naught remains but to bid you God-speed. Au revoir, mes Amis. Auf Wiedersehen, meine Brüder. Fare thee well, O most excellent English host. We thrill with pride at the achievements of the Mother country. May God prosper us all and grant that we may meet again after four years in beautiful Munich (1).

Four years later, the First World War was in its third year, and the world congress of neurology in Munich was never held. Medicine had grown to such a scale that world congresses of medicine now had to focus on specialized aspects.

The International Congress of Psychiatry, Neurology, Psychology and Care of the Insane (Amsterdam 1907)

The first International Congress of Psychiatry, Neurology, Psychology, and Care of the Insane took place in Amsterdam in September 1907. Epilepsy was a central topic for the three disciplines. International congresses for the Care and Treatment of the Insane had been held as early as 1900 and 1906. An international epilepsy organization—the concept of the International League Against Epilepsy (ILAE)—had been proposed in 1906, but the idea did not materialize until 1909. ILAE was founded on 29 August 1909 in Budapest, and had its fourth meeting in London, 1913, in conjunction with the International Congress of Medicine. It has since evolved into a global professional organization, and stimulated a global lay organization, the International Bureau for Epilepsy (IBE).

The schism between traditional psychiatry, which to a great extent was asylum based, and the supporters of Freudian psychoanalysis, was deep, although differences of opinion were only half-heartedly expressed in Amsterdam.

The First International Neurological Congress (Berne, 1931)

The first international neuroscience meeting took place in Berne, Switzerland, in September 1931 (2) (Fig. 1.1). Bernard Sachs (1858–1944) was the Congress President, Sir Charles Sherrington (1857–1952) Vice President and Henry Alsop Riley (1887–1966) the Secretary-General. The Congress, which was a result of a generous initiative by the American Neurological Association, brought together individuals from 42 countries on four continents.

There was no world organization of neurology. The idea of an international neurology meeting was born in 1927, when two neurologists, Bernard Sachs and Otto Marburg (1874–1948), met in Bad Gastein, an Austrian spa town, and discussed the needs for neurologists to come together to discuss neurosciences

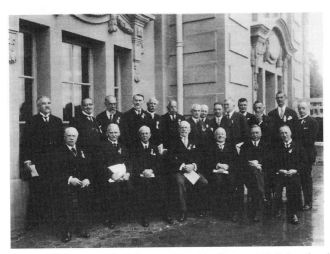

Fig. 1.1 The First International Neurological Congress (Berne, 1931). Bernhard Sachs (seated fourth from left), Otto Marburg (standing third from left).

Reproduced from Elan D. Louis. The conceptualization and organization of the first International Neurological Congress (1931): the coming of age of neurology. *Brain* 2010 133(7) 2160–66 Fig. 1. © The Author (2010). Published by Oxford University Press on behalf of the Guarantors of *Brain*.

and progress in neurology. The following year, Bernard Sachs, who was the Vice President of the American Neurological Association, wrote to key figures in international neurology, proposing an international neurological congress to be held in the late summer of 1929.

According to Gordon Holmes (1876–1965) 'the only difficulty may be to get the French and Germans to mix'. It was the first time since the World War of 1914–1918 that neurologists from former enemy countries had found it possible to have a joint meeting. Mikhail B. Kroll (1879–1939) participated as Chairman of the Soviet Delegation and represented the new Soviet nation.

But the political international unrest was much more generalized than being only European. The delegate from Argentina, Adolfo M. Sierra, wrote to Riley:

> Due to the political events that have shaken my country, from the month of September 1930, I was unable to handle the affairs of the International Neurological Congress. I had to stay away from my country for some time. The revolution that took place in my Country at that date brought new people to the scientific and political lead of Argentina. I personally, for the reasons indicated, cannot continue to preside in my office as it relates to the next Congress in Berne.
>
> It is my understanding, Dr. Henry Alsop Riley, that you have to address directly the present president of the Executive committee of the Fourth National Congress of Medicine. Prof. Jose Arce would be the man in Argentina to designate the members of the Argentinian Commission for the next International Neurological Congress. Professor Jose Arce is a member of the new Government and could be very useful to you. I urge you, Sir, to write to him as soon as possible.

In Germany, neurology was still not recognized as a separate specialty. German neurologists were grouped together with the psychiatrists in the Gesellschaft Deutscher Nervenärzte, and there were relatively few German neurologists at the meeting. Another reason why so few German neurologists attended the congress was the internal situation in Germany: the country had severe economic and political problems.

The Berne congress was important because it was one of the first occasions for neurologists from different countries to meet, learn from each other, and exchange views. But the idea of organizing a worldwide club of neurological societies was still 25 years away (2). Before World War II, the journey by sea across the Atlantic usually took about five days. Progress in communication would be necessary for the future development of international neurology.

The Second International Neurological Congress (London 1935)

Neurologists again met four years later, this time in London, in July 1935. Gordon Holmes was President and Bernard Sachs Honorary President. Samuel

Alexander Kinnier Wilson (1878–1937) was the Secretary-General. The congress was held in the large hall of University College, Gower Street. Gordon Holmes had to substitute for Sir Charles Sherrington, who had had to withdraw on health grounds. Macdonald Critchley (1900–1997), then a junior colleague of Kinnier Wilson and Gordon Holmes, described them as the two supreme figures among the world's neurologists in the 1920s and 1930s.

The official languages at the congress were English, French, German, Italian, and Spanish. However, if anyone wanted to present his communications in Italian or Spanish, they had had to forward an abstract of the paper either in English, French, or German (3).

The congress coincided with the centenary of the birth of John Hughlings Jackson (1835–1911). Kinnier Wilson had been one of Jackson's last house physicians at the National Hospital, Queen Square, from 1904 until Jackson retired in 1906. The main theme, appropriately for the Jackson jubilee, was the epilepsies. William G. Lennox (1884–1960) introduced a new chapter in epilepsy research by applying Berger's recently discovered human electroencephalograph (EEG) in 31 patients. He had demonstrated abnormal electrical changes prior to seizures. Wilder Penfield (1891–1976) had applied the EEG and cortical stimulation to demonstrate the new possibilities for epilepsy surgery in patients with focal cortical atrophy and scars (4).

Other themes were the physiology and pathology of the cerebrospinal fluid; the functions of the frontal lobe; and the hypothalamus and central representation of the autonomic nervous system. A distinguished guest at the London congress was Ivan Pavlov (1849–1936), now in his 87th year, who was honoured by an editorial in the *Lancet*.

The London congress was central to the rise of lobotomy. Carlyle Jacobsen (1902–1974) and John Farquhar Fulton (1899–1960) reported on behavioural changes, which they had observed in chimpanzees after frontal lobe lesions. Following the presentation, Egas Moniz (1874–1955), from Lisbon (Portugal), arose and suggested that it might be feasible to relieve anxiety states in man by surgical means. The following year, Egas Moniz and the Portuguese neurosurgeon Pedro Almeida Lima (1903–1985) presented the first results of lobotomy in human psychotic patients. Walter Freeman (1895–1972), an American neurologist, had also attended the London congress, where he had met with Egas Moniz. They formed a strong professional relationship. Freeman reported on his first lobotomy in 1936 (5).

The official organ of the ILAE, *Epilepsia*, had ceased to exist after the outbreak of the First World War. At the end of the London congress, delegates came together at the Lingfield colony in London and agreed to re-establish and reconstitute the ILAE and the journal, and elected William Lennox as President (3).

The Third International Neurological Congress (Copenhagen 1939)

The Congress took place in Copenhagen, Denmark, from 21 to 25 August 1939. The Munich agreement on Czechoslovakia was in September 1938. Italy had invaded Albania in April 1939. Germany had announced the annexation of Austria in March 1939. In a telegram to Adolf Hitler, 14 April 1939, President Franklin Delano Roosevelt wrote:

> Throughout the world hundreds of millions of human beings are living today in constant fear of a new war or even a series of wars.

In view of the doubt expressed by some Americans as to the advisability of holding the congress in Denmark, neighbouring Germany, some American neurologists communicated with the Danish congress committee requesting their opinion. The Danish committee replied that they believed it advisable to continue with the plans for the congress and that if present conditions continued, the congress would be held in Copenhagen, as already determined.

One week after the congress had ended, World War II began with the invasion of Poland by Germany and subsequent declarations of war on Germany by France and most of the countries of the British Empire and Commonwealth. Attendance at the congress was, however, remarkably good, although the *Lancet* commented that the contingent from Great Britain was smaller than it would have been in more settled times.

The opening of the congress was in the large assembly hall at the University of Copenhagen. Professor Viggo Christiansen (1867–1939) was the President, Gordon Holmes, Bernhard Sachs, and Sir Charles Sherrington Honorary Presidents. There were no fewer than 11 Vice Presidents, among them Ludo van Bogaert (1897–1989), who later became the first President of the World Federation of Neurology. Knud Krabbe was Secretary-General. The main topics of the congress were the autonomic nervous system, heredo-familiar disorders, and neurological aspects of the avitaminoses, with special reference to the peripheral nervous system. There was also a full day devoted to neurosurgery, the first truly international neurosurgical meeting. The international ILAE meeting took place during the congress, and there was an excursion to the Epileptics Hospital at Dianalund (6).

One central issue during this congress was the introduction of electroconvulsive therapy (ECT) in psychiatry. Professor Lucio Bini (1908–1964) reported on the use of electricity to induce seizures for therapeutic purposes in psychiatric patients. This was the first presentation of ECT before a large international audience, and it spread rapidly within the world of psychiatry (7).

The Fourth International Neurological Congress (Paris 1949)

The Second World War put a virtual stop to international meetings. Plans had been made for a congress to be held in Paris in 1943 but they were not realized until 1949. At an EEG meeting at the National Hospital for Nervous Diseases in Queen Square, London, UK, in 1947, the American neurophysiologist Wladimir Theodore Liberson (1904–1994) stated:

> There is no problem more significant in its implications for peace, for international solidarity, for cultural co-operation, than the study of the brain.

The Fourth International Neurological Congress was held in Paris in September 1949. Théophile Alajouanine was the President, and Raymond Garcin was Secretary-General. The four main topics selected for discussion were the thalamus and its pathology; electroencephalography and electromyography; virus diseases of the nervous system; neurosurgery, especially cordotomy and psychosurgery. During the meeting, Alfonso Asenjo (Chile) organized a minor meeting for neurosurgeons to discuss the presentation of neurosurgery at future international congresses.

The first International EEG Congress (founding meeting) had taken place in London in 1947, and the organizers wanted the Second International EEG Congress to get into step with the neurological congress which was to be held in Paris two years later. This congress focused upon EEG, but the final day was a joint one where one of the topics was electromyography.

The number of free communications submitted for the scientific sessions had increased to an alarming degree, and also posed a problem of increased costs for the publication of transactions and projection equipment. At the end of the Congress, a liaison committee was appointed to bind the interests of these groups more closely to those of neurology (8).

The congress coincided with the centenary of the birth of Joseph Jules Dejerine (1849–1917), and the participants could attend a lecture at the Sorbonne by André Thomas (1867–1963), who gave a discourse on Dejerine's life and achievements. There were 1440 active participants from 46 different countries, and 199 of the enrolled were Americans, not unexpectedly the largest number (9).

The Fifth International Congress of Neurological Sciences (Lisbon, 1953)

The fifth congress of neurology was held in Lisbon in September 1953, and was followed by a meeting in Madrid to commemorate the centenary of the birth of Ramon y Cajal (1852–1934).

The President of the Congress was António Flores, and Pedro Almeida Lima was Secretary-General. Honorary Presidents were Gordon Holmes, Georges Charles Guillain (1876–1961), André Thomas, Théophile Alajouanine (1890–1980), and Egas Moniz.

There were two sessions on cerebrovascular conditions, by Moniz and by Alajouanine. Sir Francis Walshe (1885–1973) discussed the functions of the parietal lobe, and Ludo van Bogaert reviewed metabolic diseases of the nervous system. The ILAE meeting took place following the congress. It was a one-day meeting on temporal lobe epilepsies, and the discussion placed temporal lobe epilepsy at the centre of contemporary clinical and research interest. The meeting was conceived and convened by Henri Gastaut, the new ILAE President-elect, who had devoted all his activities in the previous five years to the study of the temporal epilepsies (10).

Briefly, the Lisbon Congress demonstrated (1) a lack of cooperation on the part of some authors who presented their papers late or not at all because they considered their audiences too small and unworthy of them; (2) the crushing weight of the increasing number of free communications which evoked relatively little interest; (3) the failure of holding many small sessions devoted to free communications compared with the success of large symposia; and (4) the susceptibility of national pride when selection of authors was made, which hampered the freedom of a topic director to choose his own collaborators (11).

The First International Congress of Neurological Sciences—the Sixth International Neurological Congress (Brussels July 21–28, 1957)

The congress took place in Brussels. Paul van Gehuchten was President and Ludo van Bogaert Secretary-General. Sir Gordon Holmes, Georges Charles Guillain, André Thomas, Théophile Alajouanine, António Flores, Georg H. Monrad-Krohn (Norway), Knud Krabbe (Denmark), Henry Alsop Riley (USA), and Paul Divry were Honorary Presidents.

Why was this 'the Sixth International Neurological Congress'? The First International Neurological Congress was held in Berne in 1931, and subsequent meetings had taken place in London, Copenhagen, Paris, and Lisbon. It therefore became the Sixth International Congress of Neurology. The International League Against Epilepsy had been formed in 1907, and this association was due to hold its international conference. The year 1957 was also the time for the Third International Congress of Neuropathology, the Fifth Congress of Neuroradiology, and the Fourth International Congress of Electroencephalography and Clinical Neurophysiology; for the first time there was also an International

Congress of Neurosurgery. But this was a topic under discussion. Sir Francis Walshe was critical of a joint congress: 'Do not desert us now, neurology is at the cross-road'. The neurosurgeon Sir Geoffrey Jefferson commented dryly, 'Where else has it ever been?' It had been discussed whether to have neurosurgery as one of the scientific topics during the Lisbon congress, but the proposal received only partial support. The plurality of several international congresses of neurosciences is one of the reasons why the Brussels congress in 1957 was also named the First International Congress of Neurological Sciences (10).

The Congress was held at the Palais des Beaux Arts de Bruxelles. The combined formal opening took place on Sunday 21 July in the late afternoon, in the presence of His Majesty the King and members of the Belgian Government.

After a musical overture, the presidents of the various neuroscience organizations participating in the congress delivered brief addresses of welcome. They were then introduced to the King of Belgium, who extended greetings and wishes for a successful congress. Approximately 2000 persons attended the congress, of whom about half were neurologists. The largest contingents came from Great Britain, the USA, France, and Germany, but the international nature of the meeting was upheld by members from Chile and Japan, from Venezuela and Yugoslavia, from Poland and Peru. The congress was well organized, but some individuals—not only EEG doctors—felt lost and were afraid the intimacy of the previous congress had gone forever (11).

This year also witnessed the centenary of the births of Charles Sherrington, Victor Horsley, and Joseph Babinski, to whom homage was paid respectively by Raymond Garcin (France), Ernest Sachs (Newhaven, USA), and Sir Geoffrey Jefferson (UK).

A joint meeting of all the disciplines, dedicated to the memory of Sir Charles Sherrington and devoted to the study of extrapyramidal pathology, was held under the directorship of Raymond Garcin. Modern surgical methods in the treatment of Parkinsonism were reviewed, particularly the destructive procedures directed to the globus pallidus.

There was a plenary session on multiple sclerosis and demyelinating diseases under the chairmanship of Houston Merritt and opened by Georg H. Monrad-Krohn. Experimental allergic encephalomyelitis was a relatively new concept in 1957, and nobody had yet produced multiple sclerosis in the experimental animal. Many papers were devoted to the experimental production of demyelination. It was reported that the level of gamma globulin is raised in the active phases of multiple sclerosis and that the level can be reduced to normal by giving corticotropin. One claim was made that ACTH given over a period of three years might have some therapeutic effect, and a similar claim was made for repeated blood transfusions.

Although the Brussels congress was excellent, its main importance was its effect upon the planning of a future world organization of neurology.

References

1 **Monrad-Krohn GH.** Et tilbakeblikk. *T Norske Lægeforen* 1964; **84**(5): 451–76.

2 **Louis E.** The conceptualization and organization of the first International Neurological Congress (1931): the coming of age of neurology. *Brain* 2010; **133**(7): 2160–6.

3 **Wilson SAK.** Report on the conference of the programme-executive committee of the second international neurological congress, London 1935. *J Neuro Psychopathol* 1934; s1–14: 283–8.

4 **Bladin PF.** The threshold of the new epileptology: Dr. Lennox at the London Congress, 1935. *J Clin Neurosci* 2010; **17**(1): 16–21.

5 **Shorter E.** The Lobotomy Adventure. In Shorter E, Ed., *A History of Psychiatry*. John Wiley & Sons, New York 1997, pp 225–9.

6 **Finland IF.** Third International Neurological Congress, Copenhagen 1939. *Acta Psychiat Scand* 1938; **13**(3): 327–35.

7 **Kragh JV.** The origins of electroconvulsive therapy in Denmark. *J ECT* 2009; **25**(4): 270–3.

8 **Fourth International Neurological Congress 1949.** *Br Med J* 1949; **2** (4629): 697–8.

9 **Shorvon S.** An Episode in the History of Temporal Lobe Epilepsy: The Quadrennial Meeting of the ILAE in 1953. *Epilepsia* 2006; **47**(8): 1288–91.

10 **Nuwer MR, Lücking CH.** Wave length and action potentials: History of the International Federation of Clinical Neurophysiology. *Clin Neurophysiol* 2010; **61**(Suppl): 1–280.

11 **Congress of Neurological Sciences.** From a special correspondent. *Br Med J* 17 August 1957.

Chapter 2

The Shaping of the Organization

It is imperative that a world federation of neurological
societies be established to replace the presently existing
system of organization of international congresses based
on convenience and individual friendship. This world
federation would elect officers who would act as liaison
with the allied disciplines, two of which have already
constituted a federation.
(Ludo van Bogaert)

The World Federation of Neurology (WFN) was born in Brussels in July 1957,
during the First International Congress of Neurological Sciences (Sixth International Neurological Congress). Ludo van Bogaert was elected President,
Macdonald Critchley and Auguste Tournay, Vice Presidents, and Pearce Bailey,
Secretary-Treasurer General.

How did it start, and who were the movers?

The original idea of the WFN arose during a dinner in Antwerp in 1955. Van
Bogaert, Armand Lowenthal, and Charles Poser (then at the Institute Bunge as
a Fulbright scholar), discussed the formation of a club consisting mainly of neuropathologists (named were Christensen, Löken, Scholz, Hallervorden, Spatz,
Schaltenbrand, Bertrand, Gruner) and some neurologists (Critchley, Garcin,
Monrad-Krohn). The purpose was primarily to collect reprints and unpub-
lished doctoral theses in a central location (e.g. the Institute Bunge). As the
discussion progressed, they thought that the group should be expanded and
that other specialists should also form such 'clubs'.

From there, many other talks occurred. By the time Poser left, in June 1955,
the concept had evolved of a world federation involving all specialists in neurology. In the meanwhile, the federation was discussed more thoroughly with a
number of prominent neurologists, but the main supporters were Houston

Merritt, Pearce Bailey, and Macdonald Critchley. Invitations were sent for a founding meeting in 1957.

Was there a need among neurologists to form an international organization? Twelve years had passed since World War II. There was a gulf between European and American neurology.

Medical neurology had undergone a renaissance in the USA after World War II. The personal efforts of Pearce Bailey, Houston Merritt, and Abe Baker had been instrumental in this respect, also for international collaboration. The American Academy of Neurology, and its journal *Neurology*, had been initiated ten years before the birth of the WFN. The establishment of the National Institute of Neurological Diseases and Blindness (NINDB), with its Federal support, was extremely important, not least because of the generous support to the WFN during the critical start period. The outcome of these circumstances is reflected in the dominant position occupied by the USA on the international neurological scientific scene.

Both clinical and scientific training and collaboration had changed. American neurologists occasionally studied in Europe, most of them at the National Hospital for Nervous Diseases at Queen Square in London. According to Charles Poser, continental European neurology consisted of a tightly knit club, led by physicians who had learned clinical neurology at the Salpêtrière in Paris, many of them also with a background in neuropathology from Spielmeyer's laboratory in Munich. Communication was slow, international travelling expensive and complicated, and language problems difficult. Neurology also flourished outside Europe and North America (examples were Argentina, Australia, Japan, and India), but international contacts were few. In other medical specialties, the need for collaboration had been realized, and an international organization had already been established for electroencephalographs. Why not for neurology?

The movers were two Americans and one European, Houston Merritt, Pearce Bailey, and Ludo van Bogaert. Ludo van Bogaert (1897–1989) from Antwerp, Belgium, was the leading neuropathologist of his time, and also a respected neurologist. Houston Merritt and Pearce Bailey had already proposed the creation of a world neurological federation at the meeting of the American Academy of Neurology in 1956, and the proposal had been approved unanimously.

Merritt had visited Antwerp and knew that plans had been made for a First International Congress of the Neurological Sciences, and that it should take place in 1957. Preliminary meetings for this congress were held in Brussels in 1955. It was meant to be a single venue for neurology, neuropathology, neurosurgery, clinical neurophysiology, and neuroradiology (1, 2).

Houston Merritt (1902–1979) was one of the most respected clinical neurologists in the USA. He was the Director of the Neurological Institute of the Columbia Presbyterian Medical Center in New York from 1948 to 1967. He was also the Dean of the Columbia University College of Physicians and Surgeons from 1958 to 1969.

H. Houston Merritt (1902–1979)

This section was written by Lewis P. Rowland.

Houston Merritt must have been one of the most unassuming world leaders in any field. He was born in Wilmington, NC, and considered himself 'a barefoot boy'. But when he died, obituaries in several medical journals (1) and one book about him and his research partner, Tracy Putnam, placed him securely among the great neurologists of all time. His crowning achievement was the discovery of phenytoin (diphenylhydantoin or Dilantin), an anticonvulsant that led the way to the discovery of newer drugs.

He attended the University of North Carolina and Vanderbilt University before his medical training at Johns Hopkins. He later received honorary degrees from Harvard, New York Medical College, and Columbia University. After training in medicine at New Haven Hospital, he went to the Boston City Hospital as neurology resident. In 1930, he studied neuropathology in Germany and then returned to Boston for a 13-year career at Harvard, culminating as an Associate Professor of Neurology.

In 1944, Dr Merritt became a Professor of Clinical Neurology at Columbia University and Chief of the Division of Neuropsychiatry at Montefiore Hospital. After four years, he became Chairman of the Department of Neurology at Columbia and director of the Neurological Service at the Neurological Institute of the Presbyterian Hospital in New York. In 1958, he was appointed Dean of the College of Physicians and Surgeons. As Dean, he supervised revision of the curriculum, increased the number of women and minority students, started an affiliation with Harlem Hospital, and had a research building constructed. He retired as Chairman in 1967 and as Dean in 1970.

His contributions were recorded in 215 scientific papers and five books on cerebrospinal fluid, epilepsy, neurosyphilis, headache, stroke, multiple sclerosis, and genetic diseases. As neurological research became more diverse and more sophisticated, Merritt sponsored research in his own department and as an official advisor to the NINDB in Bethesda, MD, serving on the National Advisory Council for that Institute from 1950 to 1964. At a time when neurology was being overshadowed by the success of neurosurgery and psychiatry, Merritt was influential in the emergence of modern neurology. He was a leader in the maturation of voluntary health agencies for muscular dystrophy, multiple sclerosis, cerebral palsy, Parkinsonism, epilepsy, and myasthenia gravis. His awards were numerous and his influence was international.

He was Vice President of the Sixth International Congress (Brussels, 1955), the Seventh Congress (Rome, 1961), and the Eighth Congress (Vienna, 1965). He was President of the Ninth Congress, which was held in New York City in 1969. He was an honorary member of societies in London, France, Argentina, and those in Philadelphia and Chicago. He was given the title of Officer of the Portuguese Order of Santiago for his care of António de Oliveira Salazar. In addition to these international efforts, Merritt was one of the founders of the World Federation of Neurology.

One of Houston Merritt's notable achievements actually increased his influence. Among the roughly 100 medical schools in the USA, students of Houston Merritt have been leaders of more than 30 departments of neurology. Joseph Foley, one of his trainees, called Merritt 'Neurologist to the world'.

Pearce Bailey (1902–1976) was the Director of the National Institutes of Health (NIH) in Bethesda, MD. He was fluent in French, an ability that was important in the new situation.

Pearce Bailey, Junior (1902–1976)

This section was written by Lewis P. Rowland.

The second neurologist named Pearce Bailey came on the scene at a more opportune time than his father. That is, the establishment of the NINDB in 1950 was a milestone in the history of neurology in the USA. Money became available for research, including the training of young investigators at a time when there were few. Funds also became available to support independent researchers. Among those who came to the NIH for research training were many who returned to the medical schools where they had been educated. In the process, elite schools prospered and funds became available throughout the country to open new programmes.

According to one estimate, 'neurologically disabled veterans in the post-war years accounted for about 25 percent of the patients in general hospitals and 10 percent of those in psychiatric hospitals.' In addition, about 1.7 million men had been rejected for military service because of a neuropsychiatric condition or a learning disorder.

The NIH started with the establishment of the National Cancer Institute in 1937, followed by the Heart Institute in 1948. In 1948 the American Academy of Neurology was also created. Advocacy groups promoted research for multiple sclerosis, cerebral palsy, muscular dystrophy, epilepsy, and blindness. The paucity of clinical neurologists or research neuroscientists became evident. The support of public leaders like Mary Lasker and Senator Claude Pepper stimulated public and Congressional awareness. The time was right for a neurological institute at the NIH.

In 1951, Pearce Bailey Jr., was appointed the first Director of NINDB (3). He was a graduate of Princeton, had an MA degree from Columbia, and a PhD from the University of Paris (Sorbonne). He was associate director of the Psychological Centre in Paris from 1933 to 1936, returned to the USA for medical training at the Medical College of South Carolina, and was trained in Neurology on the Cornell division at Bellevue Hospital (3). He then served as chief of the neurology service at the Philadelphia Naval Hospital. He became head of the Neurology Section of the Veterans Administration (VA) Central Office in 1946. He returned to Europe in 1959 as director of international research for NINDS in Antwerp, Belgium. In 1962 he led international research programmes in Puerto Rico.

He had been Chief of Neurology for the Veterans Administration, where he had supervised the development of programmes for patient care as well as clinical and research training. He guided the national programme that affiliated each VA hospital to a medical school. He was also one of the founders of the newly minted American Academy of Neurology in 1948 and was the second president of that organization in 1949–50. It was a busy time for him.

In 1951, Bailey wrote the first article published on page 1 of the first issue of *Neurology*, the official journal of the Academy. The journal was destined to become a major force in the development of neurology worldwide.

Bailey made two important choices at high levels of administration. First, he picked Seymour Kety to lead the intramural research programmes, with laboratories on the NIH campus in Bethesda, Maryland. As a result of Kety's insight, 20 of the investigators appointed to be laboratory chiefs in NINDB or NIMH were ultimately elected to the National Academy of Sciences, one of the highest honours for a researcher in the USA.

Bailey also made a brilliant choice in appointing G. Milton Shy as Intramural Clinical Director of NINDB in 1953, when the NIH research hospital opened. Shy was the founder of modern research in neuromuscular diseases and other conditions, including one that bears his name, the Shy–Drager syndrome. In turn, Shy appointed W. King Engel, who complemented Shy's efforts. Shy was only 33 years old when he was chosen 'on grounds of promise'.

Among the achievements of NINDB were 'field studies' that were conducted in Guam and Maracaibo in remote Venezuela. D. Carleton Gajdusek and C. Joseph Gibbs, who provided evidence that chronic brain disease could be caused by virus-like agents, led the Guam research on transmissible diseases. Ultimately, this work established the existence of prions. The Venezuelan research set an epidemiological approach to a genetic disease. These and other NINDB programmes were awarded five Lasker Awards and six Nobel Prizes.

Dr Bailey was surely an international figure. He was Secretary-Treasurer General of the World Federation of Neurology (1959–65) and was an honorary member of neurological societies in Argentina, Rio de Janeiro, Montevideo, Japan, Peru, Greece, France, Germany and New York.

Behind the scenes: a preliminary meeting in Brussels

Before the congress, letters of invitation had been sent to national neurological societies throughout the world that there would be an organizational meeting during the congress, and invited them to send a delegate (Fig. 2.1). Fortunately, international neurology was outside politics, and representatives from the USSR, Bulgaria, Czechoslovakia, Hungary, Poland, and Romania attended the Brussels meeting and could mingle with colleagues from the West.

These were the 38 national delegates who met in Brussels: Roman Arana-Iñiguez (Uruguay), Alfonso Asenjo (Chile), Pearce Bailey (USA), Juan José Barcia Goyanes (Spain), G. Belloni (Italy), Sam Berman (South Africa), S. Bojinov

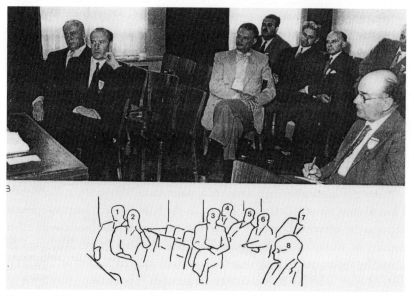

Fig. 2.1 Behind the scenes: a preliminary meeting in Brussels. Organizational meeting of the WFN, Brussels 26 July 1957.

1. Sükrü Aksel (Turkey), 2. Macdonald Critchley (UK), 3. G. Wohlfart (Sweden), 4. Bojinov (Bulgaria), 5. G. Usunov (Bulgaria), 6. E. Herman (Poland), 7. G. Schaltenbrand (Germany), 8. G. Belloni (Italy).

Reprinted from *J Neurol. Sci*, 120, C. Poser, The World Federation of Neurology: the formative period. Personal recollections 1955 – 1961, 218–227. Copyright (1993), with permission from Elsevier.

(Bulgaria), C. Castell-Diaz (Uruguay), Deolindo Couto (Brazil), Macdonald Critchley (UK), C. de Rojas (Cuba), J. Espadaler Medina (Spain), R. Frauchiger (Switzerland), Nikolai Grashchenkov (USSR), Leo Halpern (Israel), Kamil Henner (Czechoslovakia), E. Herman (Poland), Knud Krabbe (Denmark), S. Kornyev (Hungary), A. Kreindler (Romania), Erik Kugelberg (Sweden), J.Lopez-Ibor (Spain), Houston Merritt (USA), Georg H. Monrad-Krohn (Norway), S. Nachev (Bulgaria), José Pereyra-Käfer (Argentina), B. Ramamurthi (India), Sigvald Refsum (Norway), Georg Schaltenbrand (W. Germany), M. Sercl (Czechoslovakia), C. Sillevis-Smitt (the Netherlands), Ihsan Sükrü Aksel (Turkey), E. Tchehrazi (Iran), Auguste Tournay (France), Oscar Montes Trelles (Peru), Knud Winther (Denmark), Gunnar Wohlfart (Sweden), N. Zec (Yugoslavia)

The delegates represented 29 national societies, 19 of them European, six Latin American (Argentina, Brazil, Chile, Cuba, Peru, Uruguay). There were two neurologists from the USA (Bailey and Merritt), one from Africa (South Africa) and two from Asia (Iran and India) (5).

The meetings took place 22 and 26 July 1957. Ludo van Bogaert (Antwerp, Belgium) was unanimously elected President of the new organization. Pearce Bailey (Bethesda, USA) became Secretary-Treasurer General.

Four Vice Presidents of the WFN were elected, Houston Merritt, Raymond Garcin, Kamil Henner, and Shigeo Okinaka. Van Bogaert, Merritt, Critchley, Tournay, Schaltenbrand, and Bailey had prepared a draft for a constitution. An informal WFN Policy Committee was formed to consider the future policy of the new organization. It consisted of WFN members from different countries. Among them were Macdonald Critchley, Eddie P. Bharucha (Bombay, India), Russell N. DeJong (Ann Arbor, USA), Georg Schaltenbrand (West Germany), Francois Thiébaut (Strasbourg, France), Oscar Montes Trelles (Lima, Peru), and Semen Aleksandrovich Sarkisov (Moscow, USSR). Because the term policy had different meanings in different countries, the Policy Committee was renamed the Steering Committee in 1969 (5, 6).

Ludo van Bogaert: the formative years

Ludovicus (Ludo) Maria Carolus Gommarus van Bogaert was born in Antwerp on 25 May 1897 into an ancient family with liberal but nevertheless Catholic convictions and undeniable Flemish roots (Fig. 2.2). His father and his younger brother Adalbert (1904–96) were both physicians. When World War I broke out in 1914, Ludo van Bogaert volunteered for the army, but was not accepted because of his young age. He then took the preparatory courses for medicine, and joined the Belgian army in France in 1916. He was wounded twice, most

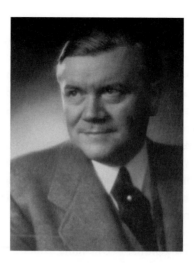

Fig. 2.2 Ludo van Bogaert, the first WFN President—the formative years.

Courtesy of Erik Baeck.

severely in September 1918, when a machine-gun bullet pierced his right lung and damaged the spine, resulting in a temporary paralysis of both legs.

He enrolled at the Faculté de Médecine of the Université Libre de Bruxelles in January 1919, obtained his medical degree with the highest honours in July 1922, and decided to go to Paris to specialize. He worked at the Salpêtrière with Professor Pierre Marie, and at the laboratory of Professor Marcel Labbé at the Hôpital de la Charité, and returned in 1923. He defended his thesis on 'Les lesions cérébrales dans la sclérose amyotrophique' in 1925.

Ludo van Bogaert had met and worked with several of the leading neuropathologists in the 1920s, such as Brouwer and Ariens in Amsterdam, von Economo in Vienna, von Monakow in Zürich, and in the Vogt laboratories in Berlin.

Van Bogaert was a neuropathologist, but also a clinician. He had taken over his late father's private practice in Antwerp, and in 1923 was appointed 'additional-doctor' in the Department of Internal Medicine at Stuyvenberg Hospital, where he established a laboratory of histopathology. From 1934 to 1949 he acted as head of the Department of Internal Medicine at Stuyvenberg Hospital for '2 hours a day, 6 days a week and 52 weeks a year'. In 1930, van Bogaert married Marie-Louis Sheid, daughter of an Antwerp ship-owner. They moved to a magnificent patrician home in Antwerp. The marriage remained childless.

In 1934, the Bunge Institute was formally opened. It was founded in memory of Edouard Bunge (1851–1927), who was president–director of a worldwide trading company in Antwerp. Edouard Bunge wanted to establish a Centre of Medical and Surgical Research where complete diagnostic examinations as well as scientific investigations could be combined. Ludo van Bogaert became the head of the Department of Internal Medicine and Neurology, but before the official inauguration of the new institute, 4 July 1934, he had already transferred his laboratory from Stuyvenberg Hospital to the new location where, on 1 February 1934, he opened the Section of Anatomopathology with assistance from Dr H-J. Scherer. His brother, Adalbert van Bogaert, became the head of the Laboratory of Experimental Medicine.

The institute soon became internationally known. Young scientists from all over the world were given the opportunity to work in the laboratories of the Bunge Institute. The main scientific papers were published biannually in *Travaux de l'Institut Bunge*. In 1937, Ludo van Bogaert received a donation from the Rockefeller Foundation. In 1938, the establishment of a Fund of Dotation and Research from the Born family supported the Bunge Institute.

In 1967, the Foundation Born–Bunge and the Rijksuniversitaire Centrum Antwerpen formed a partnership, and in 1977 the laboratories of the Born–Bunge Foundation were transferred to the campus of the Universitaire Instelling Antwerpen. Although the Born–Bunge Foundation kept its autonomy, the Neurological Department of the Bunge Institute, which closed in 1979, was integrated into the newly built university hospital at Edegem. The closing of the Bunge Institute meant the end of van Bogaert's career, but his scientific heritage remained in Antwerp. Currently, the Born–Bunge Institute is still active but is integrated into the University of Antwerp.

Ludo van Bogaert authored 753 publications, with 175 as first author. He described several neurological disorders with detailed descriptions of the neuropathology. He covered nearly all the fields of clinical and animal neuropathology, but his main field of interest was hereditary metabolic and degenerative diseases, especially the lipidoses. He represented the best of the classical European tradition with a combination of clinical and neuropathological expertise. Ludo van Bogaert could have been professor at the Université Libre de Bruxelles, but he refused the prerequisite of denying his Catholic faith (13). He received, however, the insignia of *doctoris honoris causa* from several universities (Utrecht, Montpellier, Freiburg im Breisgau, Genève, Liège, Lyon, Tübingen, Sienna). In 1962, King Baudouin raised van Bogaert to a barony.

In 1957, he was the Secretary-General of the First International Congress of Neurological Sciences in Brussels. He was then elected first President of the WFN. He completed two terms of office (1957–1965). He also became the first President of the International Society of Neuropathology in 1968 (7–9).

The world 1957–1965: Cold War and the Wind of Change

What was happening in the world during the eight years of van Bogaert's presidency? Twelve years had passed since World War II. Europe was split by the

Iron Curtain, and the Berlin Wall was erected in 1961. There were two national German Associations of Neurology.

Nikita Krushchev was in power in the USSR, while Dwight Eisenhower was the President of the USA. John F. Kennedy took over as US President in 1961, and was assassinated in Dallas in 1963. Harold Macmillan was the British Prime Minister 1957–1963. Charles de Gaulle became French President in 1959, which meant the end of the Fourth Republic in France. The Soviet Republic dominated space science, and the first Sputnik orbited the Earth in October 1957, followed by Sputnik II one month later. Soviet intercontinental rockets were placed on Cuba. The first manned space exploration, Vostok I with Yuri Gagarin aboard, took place in 1961, and the first US astronaut, John Glenn, circled three times around the Earth. There was political unrest in North Africa; Tunis and Algeria were still colonies, and the war in the Belgian colony of Congo started in 1958. Most African countries became sovereign nations.

The world changed during these eight years. In February 1960, the British Prime Minister Harold Macmillan gave his famous speech to the South African Parliament, 'The wind of change is blowing through this continent, and whether we like it or not, this growth of national consciousness is a political fact'. This started the decolonization process in Africa. In the following years, the former colonies became independent nations.

In his Presidential Report to the World Congress of Neurology in Vienna 1965, van Bogaert was concerned about 'the two great blocks that dominate the civilized world'.

> There is no shame to admit that our Europe is but a conglomeration of small or middle-sized countries, just a province in the totality of the world. This smallness gives it a privileged position to the extent that we realize other continents are indispensable to our evolution. The destiny of Latin America, that of Asia and of Africa remains for us Europeans, essential . . . To deny the promise which we have made to assist them in their development to the limits of our power, would expose us to the risk of being engulfed in our turn by one or the other of the three hegemonies who wish to divide the world today (10).

Ludo van Bogaert's presidency

Van Bogaert was probably the only person who could pull together the various European groups and have them collaborate with the Americans and others into a World Federation of Neurology (5). He had a unique position in international neurology. His presidency became a hectic period for the new organization. The WFN had been founded, but was lacking an established international network. Even then, the specialty of neurology had a broad spectrum. There were outstanding neurologists in many countries, but they had often little or no contact with each other. The relative language barrier prevented very close contacts even between English- and French-speaking scientists. In 1957, few could foresee the explosive growth in the neurosciences and the development of new tools to understand the functions of the nervous system.

Van Bogaert's leadership was charismatic, and the WFN prospered. Most existing neurological societies became members. It was clear that the WFN, in addition to organizing quadrennial congresses, should promote international collaboration in research. This was even more important around 1960, before universities and research institutions had developed networks like they have today. Although very much a classic, French-speaking European scholar, Ludo van Bogaert had a global perspective on his work as the President of the WFN.

The WFN was founded and its first constitution and bye-laws were formulated during the First International Congress of Neurological Sciences in Brussels in 1957 (Fig. 2.3). At that time, the WFN had no budget, but the constitution provided for the billing of member societies for annual dues of $2 per member per society. Van Bogaert generously offered the facilities at the Institute Bunge for the establishment of a Central Secretariat, and made available his secretarial and professional staff.

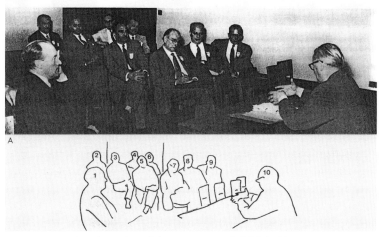

Fig. 2.3 Organizational meeting of the WFN, Brussels 26 July 1957.

1. M. Critchley (UK), 2. C. De Rojas (Cuba), 3. B. Ramamurthi (India), 4. C. Poser (USA), 5. E. Tcheazi (Iran), 6. J. Trelles (Peru), 7. G. Belloni (Italy), 8. H. Merritt (USA), 9. P. Bailey (USA), 10. L. van Bogaert (Belgium).

Reprinted from *J Neurol Sci*, 120, C. Poser, The World Federation of Neurology: the formative period. Personal recollections 1955–1961, 218–227. Copyright (1993), with permission from Elsevier.

The NIH, USA, offered an annual grant of $126,190 for five years in order to get the federation started. This gave the economic basis for an office in Antwerp ($4,662.60 for rental of office space in 1962) and the running costs to get off the ground. By the end of 1962, the WFN Secretariat had received over half a million dollars from the original NINDB grant. Some additional funds were obtained by annual subscription per active member of the national neurological societies who became members of the WFN. It soon became clear that after a few years, when the NIH seed money was gone, the funds obtained through the annual dues would be insufficient. But that was still in the future (11).

Ludo van Bogaert and Pearce Bailey organized committees of clinicians and neuroscientists with specialized interests within neurology. They were the fore-runners of the WFN Research Groups. In the following text, the original French names are preserved.

The WFN Problem Commissions

Van Bogaert and the leadership of the WFN realized the importance of creating groups of international leaders in various fields of neurology. These groups were called Problem Commissions. The Problem Commissions became very important, but they also led to the first and most dramatic internal crisis of the new organization.

The WFN was not in a position to sponsor Problem Commission meetings, which usually occurred during international congresses. In order to communicate with neurologists worldwide, an international journal was needed, and *World Neurology* was founded in 1960. The Problem Commissions published reports from their meetings in *World Neurology*, later in the *Journal of Neurological Sciences*. This formed a backbone of an international network of neurologists.

Because of the political situation in the world, and the costs of international and transatlantic journeys, many of these committees had two sections, one for the eastern and one for the western hemisphere. The major Problem Commissions had a President and a Secretary-General, sometimes with special secretaries for the eastern and the western hemisphere, respectively.

The appointed Problem Commissions reflect the world of neurology in the latter half of the 1950s more than they reflect contemporary research in the neurosciences. To some extent, they also reflect the research profiles of the founding fathers. Apparently, Parkinsonism and migraine were at that time not regarded as important problem areas in clinical neurology. Neuromuscular disorders were not included until 1964. Epilepsy was already established in another organization through the International League Against Epilepsy. During the following years, some of these Problem Commissions disappeared or were disbanded, while new ones demanded attention from the WFN.

Neuro-anatomie comparée

This had two sections. Professor Heinz Stephan chaired the eastern section, and Professor Howard A. Matzke (USA) the western. Stephan organized several symposia relevant to clinical neurology. When they met in 1965, there were 14 members and 75 corresponding members.

Neuro-anaesthesia

This was and is important. Gilbert Glaser (Montreal) was the first President; Guy Vourc´h (Paris) was chair of the eastern section, and Howard R. Terry (USA) of the western. In the absence of major financial support, Glaser and Terry recommended decentralization with two self-supporting sections. The commission was active from the beginning. It organized successful symposia, but it was soon clear that it was much more closely related to neurological surgery than to neurology. It was therefore decided in Vienna in 1963 that neuroanaesthesia should establish firm contact with the World Federation of Neurosurgical Societies (12).

Neurochimie

Armand Lowenthal, one of the WFN founders, who was an active researcher in neurochemistry, organized this Problem Commission. They met in Antwerp in September 1959. There were 12 members, and many corresponding.

Neurologie development

Stéphane Thieffry and Germaine Ribière (Paris) chaired this Problem Commission, which changed its status and function over the years.

Neurogénétique

Professor David Klein, Geneva, was founding chairman and secretary of this Problem Commission, which had its own official journal. This commission had from the beginning a close collaboration with the Problem Commission on Neuro-ophthalmologique.

Neurologie géographique, statistique et épidémique

The Problem Commission on geographic neurology, statistics and epidemiology was founded in Rome in June 1959. It reflected the importance of research on neuroepidemiological research, initially specially related to multiple sclerosis. Leonard Kurland, then Chief of the Neuroepidemiological Branch of NINDB, John Kurtzke and Kay Hyllested of Copenhagen were the founding fathers.

Maladies neuromusculaires

In 1964, John Walton proposed to the WFN President, Ludo van Bogaert, that the WFN should also have a Problem Commission on Neuromuscular Diseases. The commission was formally established in Newcastle in January 1965, and John Walton was elected Secretary and Chairman. Irena Hausmanowa-Petrusewicz of Warsaw, Christian Coërs of Brussels, Raymond Garcin of Paris, and Werner Trojaborg of Copenhagen (representing Fritz Buchtal) were present at the meeting (13).

Histoire de la Neurologie

C.D. O'Malley first chaired the Problem Commission. They organized their first symposia in Varennes in 1961 and Münster in 1962.

Neuro-oncologie

This Problem Commission, with Klaus Zülch as chairman, worked mainly to establish contacts among the members, and organized a separate symposium at the World Congress of Neurology in Vienna in 1965.

Neuro-ophthalmologique

Adolphe Francheschetti, Geneva (1896–1968), was the first Chairman and remained in that position until his death in 1968. He was also the founder and editor of the *Journal de Génétique Humaine*, and the secretary of the eastern section of the commission, while Frank W. Newell was responsible for the western hemisphere. Francheschetti organized a series of successful symposia in neuro-ophthalmology (Vienna 1964, Albi 1965, and Montreal 1967).

Paralysie cérébrale

This was a group that relatively soon disappeared from the WFN system.

Neuropathologie

Franz Seitelberger chaired this Problem Commission. *Acta Neuropathologica* in the beginning also became the official journal for the Problem Commission of Comparative Neuropathology. The WFN contributed towards the expenses of publishing. Seitelberger was the Editor-in-Chief.

Neuropathologie comparative

Professor Ernst Frauchiger, Berne, was the first Chairman and Secretary of the Problem Commission of Comparative Neuropathology, which had close contact with veterinary neuropathology.

Neuro-radiologie

No one could predict the dramatic development of neuroradiology when this Problem Commission first was formed. The first Chairman was Professor

Herrmann Fischgold (Paris). Fischgold organized Journées de Neuroradiologie in Paris in 1962, supported by the WFN. The Journées were very successful, with 250 participants. There was a discussion on side-effects of neuroradiological examinations by contrast media, how common they were, and how they could be reduced in number. It soon became clear that the development of neuroradiology necessitated an international organization for neuroradiology (14).

Rehabilitation neurologique

The Problem Commission of Neurological Rehabilitation was established in 1963. It was intended to have one group with a Secretariat in the western hemisphere and another group having their Secretariat in the eastern hemisphere, preferably in Prague under the supervision of Dr Obrda in Professor Kamil Henner's service.

Neurologie tropicale

The Problem Commission of Tropical Neurology was one of the first to be organized. It also had two sections, one for the western hemisphere (Chairman Walter E. Maffei) and one for the eastern hemisphere (Chairman Hatai Chitanwudth). At the 7th International Congress of Tropical Medicine in Rio de Janeiro in 1963, the WFN Problem Commission of Tropical Neurology had a separate symposium on atypical forms of the encephalitis. The western division of the Problem Commission established sub-commissions in Sao Paulo, Rio de Janeiro, Buenos Aires, Montevideo, and Lima. It gradually became clear that tropical neurology was such a large field of neurology that the meetings developed into International Congresses of Tropical Neurology.

In 1961, India reclaimed Goa, which had been a Portuguese colony. Noshir Wadia, who had participated in the Congress of Tropical Neurology in South America, was arrested in Lisbon on his way home, and was in a Portuguese prison in Lisbon for 2 weeks (see Chapter 8).

EEG-Neurophysiologie

This soon developed into an important area of the neurosciences.

The Problem Commission of Language Disorders was also among the first new Problem Commissions. Several colleagues objected to the name, and it was then renamed Problem Commission of Aphasiology. This commission had its first meeting at Villa Monastero, Varenna, Lake Como, 5–7 May 1966. Macdonald Critchley gave the opening speech on 'Nomenclature and definitions in aphasiology'.

The Cerebrovascular Diseases Project (CVDP)

From the very beginning, cerebrovascular disorders were regarded as an important part of neurology at the WFN. A Problem Commission of Cerebrovascular

Disease was set up, consisting of Ludo van Bogaert, Abraham Bert ('Abe') Baker (Minneapolis, USA) (1908–1988), G. Mottura (Italy), Charles Poser (WFN and USA), Sigvald Refsum (Oslo, Norway), and E. Rutishauser (Switzerland). A proposal for the research project on the geographical pathology of cerebral vascular disease was written and submitted to the NINDB, with Ludo van Bogaert as the Principal Investigator, Charles Poser Co-Principal Investigator, and Houston Merritt Financial Officer. The idea was (i) to establish methodologies for measuring atherosclerosis in cerebrovascular disease, (ii) a comparative study of the results by groups of collaborating investigators in different parts of the world using one or another of the methodologies, and (iii) a study and coordination by the principal investigator of the data and results obtained by the collaborating groups. The NINDB gave a grant of US$214,108 to fund the project.

The project started as early as 1958. During a sabbatical year at the University of Oslo in 1958, Baker became aware of an already ongoing study at the Oslo Municipal Hospital of the major cerebral blood vessels. The carotid, vertebral, and basilar arteries were sectioned in several segments, and the degree of atherosclerosis estimated. Simultaneously, similar studies were going on in Poland, France, and Strasbourg. Peter O. Yates had already established a huge project in Manchester, UK. John Moossy, a neurologist and neuropathologist at the Louisiana University in New Orleans, was invited to visit Antwerp and Oslo in August 1959 to consider the directorship of the project. Two meetings were held, in Antwerp in 1960 and in London in 1961.

The project expanded considerably. At the centre in Turin (Italy) under Drs Mottura and Stramignoni, investigations focused on the aorta, the coronaries, and the cerebral arteries, and the methods applied resembled either the one established by A. B. Baker or that by John Moossy. It gradually became clear that the WFN's function in this project was not to serve as a research institution, but as a coordinator for international collaboration.

Baker's methodology was followed at the centre in Warsaw and in Lublin and Bydgoscz, while a method applied at Pruszkow followed the one established by Yates in Manchester. The Yates methodology was introduced to the project in Paris under the direction of Paul Castaigne and Francois Lhermitte. Additional centres were established in Lima (Peru) and in Mexico. Later, Budapest and Prague also wished to participate in the project.

Several scientific papers were published, and it is unclear to what degree the investigations were coordinated in a multicentre study. It was clear that the methodologies applied differed. In his report to the WFN in 1963, Ludo van Bogaert, the Principal Investigator, concluded that it would now be wise to contemplate, when sufficient material had been collected, holding workshops for two purposes, one in Europe (Manchester) and one in the USA or in Latin America.

A series of publications resulted from this project. The final publication appeared in *Stroke* (15). Then followed the financial crisis of the WFN, which made it impossible to continue the project. From then on, there was apparently a lack of enthusiasm for what were difficult and time-consuming techniques as well as the lack of familiarity with the concept of international collaboration (5, 6, 16).

The first WFN journal: *World Neurology*

Charles Poser (Fig. 2.4) had suggested to van Bogaert in March 1959 that the WFN needed its own journal, both as a newsletter, for publication of research news, and as a forum for the Problem Commissions, announcing their meetings and reports from national and international meetings in neurology. Poser became the Editor-in-Chief, with Ludo van Bogaert and Pearce Bailey Associate Editors, and the first issue was published in July 1960.

The new journal had an ambitious programme. As the Editor-in-Chief wrote in his first editorial:

> Right from the beginning we are emphasizing the international and multilingual nature of this publication as well as the variety of the aspects of neurology which we hope to cover.
>
> World Neurology . . . requests review papers on current concepts and recent advances in their field of endeavour from authorities in clinical and basic neurology and the allied disciplines. These are then translated into English, French, German, or Spanish, in each case, a language different from the one most often used by the author. An article in any language is followed by comprehensive abstracts in the other three. (17)

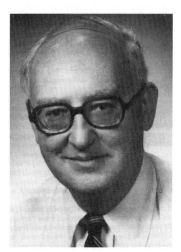

Fig. 2.4 Charles Poser.

World Neurol Vol 26. 1 February 2011. Courtesy Gustavo Roman. Copyright WFN.

Thus, Gilbert H. Glaser wrote in French on 'les cortico-stéroides et l'ACTH dans les affections nerveuses' (18), John Walton in German on 'Die progressive Muskeldystrophie—gegenwärtiger Forschungsstand' (19) and Sigvald Refsum in Spanish on 'Heredopathia atáctica polyneuritiformis. Reconsideration' (20).

Some of the papers published in *World Neurology* have remained classics in their field. In 1960, Leonard Kurland and co-workers wrote on 'Minamata Disease. The outbreak of a neurologic disorder in Minamata, Japan, and its relationship to the ingestion of seafood contaminated by mercuric compounds' (21). Pruzanski and Altman wrote on 'Encephalitis due to West Nile Fever virus' in 1962 (22). There was an epidemic in 1959 in Morocco of 10,000 cases of myelopolyneuropathy due to criminally contaminated cooking oil, which was meticulously described by Geoffroy and co-workers (23).

Seen in retrospect, publishing articles in four different languages was too ambitious and time-consuming. The Editor-in-Chief realized that standards for reviewing manuscripts varied considerably over the world. The traditions of the referee systems varied. There were considerable differences in traditions for the presentation of data, and spelling, usage, style, and grammar varied. The number of subscriptions was very slow to increase. Disagreements on editorial policy appeared. Charles Poser was replaced by Gilbert Glaser as Editor-in-Chief in September 1961, and *World Neurology* stopped publication in December 1962. It later reappeared in a totally different form as the WFN newsletter, while a new international journal was founded in 1964, still under Ludo van Bogaert's presidency. The story of the subsequent development of the new *World Neurology* will be told later.

A new journal: *Journal of the Neurological Sciences*

Ludo van Bogaert and Armand Lowenthal now negotiated a contract with Elsevier, and a new journal, *Journal of the Neurological Sciences*, official Bulletin of the World Federation of Neurology, was born in 1964, with six issues a year. Each issue contained information from the WFN with reports from committee meetings. There were also reports from meetings of national and regional neurological societies. The scientific articles had summaries in English, French, and German. Most papers were in English, but manuscripts in French or German were also accepted for publication.

In 1964, Nikolai Grashchenkov (1901–1965) urged that the journal should also accept Russian as an official language. He pointed out that there were 5000–6000 neurologists in the USSR. Van Bogaert responded that he was pleased to hear that there were so many neurologists, but this was not reflected in the dues from Russia, which amounted to US$300 (corresponding to 300 members).

THE SHAPING OF THE ORGANIZATION | **29**

Van Bogaert was sympathetic to having Russian as an official language, but pointed out that the printing costs would be too high because of the Cyrillic alphabet.

Macdonald Critchley was the first Editor-in-Chief. In 1965, he was elected President of the WFN, and John Walton became the new editor. The only financial support to the editorial office was an annual grant towards secretarial expenses of US$500 from the funds of the WFN, with no contribution from the publisher.

During the first years of its existence, the journal also served as a newsletter for the WFN. Reports from the Council of Delegates, Committee meetings, and of WFN administrative affairs were published, often occupying several pages, but not always read as thoroughly as hoped. Around 1993, when *World Neurology* had become the established WFN newsletter and published in more than 20 000 issues, the journal could focus upon its main function, being a scientific journal.

The liaison committees

During the first years of its existence, the WFN had close contact with neurosurgery, neuropathology, and electroencephalography. A Liaison Committee with neurosurgery (WFN-WFNS) was established, and met in Vienna in June 1963. For 1965, the International Congresses of Neurology and of Neurosurgery were planned for Vienna and Copenhagen respectively, and they were timed so members of the one could meet with their colleagues at the other. This arrangement was made so that the International Congress of Neuropathology to be held in Zürich took place at a convenient time for both groups. It was also decided to determine the dates and places of the congress at least five years in advance.

There was a favourable expression of opinion that other congresses of disciplines closely related to neurology and neurological surgery, i.e. EEG and Clinical Neurophysiology, Neuropathology, Epileptology, and Neuroanesthesiology be established. The Liaison Committee of the WFN and the International Federation of EEG Societies supported local meetings such as the Symposium on Electromyography, held in Copenhagen in 1963, the Marseilles Meeting, held in Cologne in 1964, and the Institution on Electroencephalography, held in Marseilles under the auspices of the WFN in 1964. The main duty of the committee was to disseminate and exchange information between neurologists and EEGs (24).

Liaison Committees with the World Psychiatric Association and the International Neuropsychological Society were established.

Over the years, however, congress participation became easier and much of this work became informal.

The WFN Decentralization Plan

> I can perfectly well understand that an agency in the USA does not wish their money to be used for the support of the administration and organizational activities of a federation situated on another continent.
> *Ludo van Bogaert, 1965*

Ludo van Bogaert and Pearce Bailey realized that in order to survive, the World Federation of Neurology had to prove that it was a true global organization. At a meeting in Cologne in 1962, a Decentralization Plan had been proposed. The principal objective was to attain a more equitable division of labour among the WFN member societies, a greater sense of participation in the total programme by the individual member societies, and a more equitable distribution of financial responsibility for the support of the WFN programme. The WFN Policy Committee convened in Vienna in 1963 during the World Congress of Neurosurgery and discussed decentralization (25).

Eddie Bharucha (India), Hans Hoff (Austria), and Russell DeJong (USA) had reservations and believed that decentralization might lead to fragmentation of the WFN and a separation of the member societies from the parent stem. A 'Committee for the Decentralization Plan' was, however, appointed under the chairmanship of Edward Graeme Robertson of Melbourne, Australia (1903–1975).

Three major regional associations were proposed, Greater European (Britain, Europe, and the USSR), Greater American (North, South, Central American, and Mexico) and the Greater Asian-Oceanian region. The regional associations would have their own secretariats, elect regional Vice Presidents and regional committees whose secretariats would be financed from regional sources. They would also serve as administrative and fiscal agents for the organization of regional and international congresses such as the First Asian-Oceanian Congress of Neurology held in Tokyo 1962, and the First Pan-American Congress of Neurology in Lima, Peru, in 1963. Both congresses were supported by grants from the NINDB.

The decentralization proposal was approved at the meeting at El Escorial in 1964 (see 'The meeting at El Escorial in May 1964', p. 32.), but not accepted as WFN decentralization. The most important consequence was the establishment of the regional organizations. In turn, they served as nuclei for the later formation of the Asian-Oceanian, the Latin American, the Pan-African, and the Pan-Arab neurological associations.

A major difficulty was the economies of centralized and decentralized secretariats. After considerable discussion, Macdonald Critchley and Ludo van Bogaert appointed a committee to be known as 'The Committee for the Decentralization Plan' to explore the matter further. The Chairman, Edward Graeme

Robertson, found that the budget for a decentralized secretariat would amount to US$3500/year, which would be the same as financing a continental secretariat. The other members were Eddie P. Bharucha (India), Shigeo Okinaka (Japan), Richard G. Robinson (New Zealand), Francois Thiébaut (France), and Román Arana-Iñiguez (Uruguay). Pearce Bailey served as Executive Secretary of this commission (25).

Rome 1961

After four hectic years, the WFN was established. The organization now had a constitution. The number of member societies had increased. Problem Commissions were focusing upon central research topics in international neurology.

In 1961, the neurologists came together for the second Congress of Neurological Sciences, in Rome this time. It was also an international congress for EEG and epilepsy, for neuropathology, and for neurosurgery, so the formal name was the 7th International Neurological Congress. The congress took place at the Palazzo Pio on the Vatican side of the river.

According to the constitution and bye-laws, the President and the Secretary-Treasurer General should each serve for four years. Ludo van Bogaert and Pearce Bailey were unanimously re-elected for a second term, and Houston Merritt and Raymond Garcin were elected Vice Presidents.

The first financial crisis of the WFN

The development of the WFN had so far been successful, but the worst was yet to come. During the second half of van Bogaert's presidency, it became clear that the organization was meeting increasing economic problems because the annual income was too low. The annual grant from the NINDB, which had been given to get the federation started, was time-limited. This fund had enabled the WFN to develop an ambitious programme for the stimulation of research and training in neurology throughout the world. Van Bogaert felt a responsibility to develop a stringent economic plan in order to rescue the organization (26, 27).

Another economic problem was that several countries had restrictions on the export of currencies. It was proposed that an account in rubles could be established in Czechoslovakia in which dues from other countries behind the Iron Curtain could be deposited. Under this arrangement it would be possible for the WFN to request funds for financing colloquiums and other WFN missions requiring expenditure in rubles. This was also approved, but the arrangement never worked.

The crisis came in the transition period between two presidents. It started during the last years of van Bogaert's presidency, but reached a climax during the first year of his successor's presidency. Economic problems now created severe problems in the organization. The WFN Policy Committee had met in Cologne in 1962 and Vienna in 1963 and discussed various ways to obtain a better distribution for the economy of the WFN programme. Van Bogaert stated that it was imperative to raise the dues from US$1.00 to US$2.00 per active member of each constituent society where this burden could be assumed without too great a hardship. The Policy Committee (26) approved this unanimously.

Ludo van Bogaert had also become sceptical about the future of the Problem Commissions. It was clear that WFN would have difficulty in financing the Problem Commissions in the future. They would receive a small amount from the WFN Secretariat for administrative expenses, but would have to apply individually for funds to support their own projects.

Ludo van Bogaert now called for a meeting of the WFN Executive Committee at El Escorial, Madrid 8–9 May 1964 (24).

The meeting at El Escorial in May 1964

The main topic was the critical economy, and how and if the WFN could avoid an economic collapse. The Secretary-Treasurer General, Pearce Bailey, described the budgetary history. He also made it clear that for 1965, the WFN would receive US$42,800 for administration and programming. After that, nothing should be expected from the NINDB for this purpose.

Van Bogaert and Bailey saw it as imperative to increase the annual member society dues from US$1 to US$2 per active member. Bailey estimated this increase to result in annual income after 1965 of approximately US$8,000 per annum. This would permit the support of a Central Secretariat at a small bookkeeping level with a secretarial staff. It would not allow for any extensive programming, travel, or the support of Problem Commissions. For that purpose, it was essential to develop a new methodology of fund-raising and/or new sources of support. The only proposal thus far to meet this emergency had been the WFN Decentralization Proposal.

Pearce Bailey then asked the assembly: 'The critical question, therefore, may be whether the WFN decentralization process continues to grow spontaneously without a clear sense of direction or whether it shall be to some degree preplanned with a sense of direction under the umbrella of the Central Secretariat whose responsibility is to integrate the decentralization elements into a harmonious whole.'

In his closing remarks, Ludo van Bogaert said: 'What disturbs me—and this is the reason for which I say that it is absolutely essential to have a decentralization plan—is that in 1965 my successor might be faced with a situation in which he would not be able to hold the World Federation together. . . . In short, I see in decentralization an undeniable necessity and one of very great need. . . . If you do not accept decentralization, I can promise you a collapse of the World Federation' (29).

The Bunge meeting December 1964: the WFN rescue plan

The situation was now becoming tense. Van Bogaert had described the three elements of his WFN rescue plan: the increase in annual dues, the decentralization plan, and the new organization for the Problem Commissions. Decisions had to be taken at the next World Congress of Neurology, in Vienna in 1965. This is why he now called for a meeting of the secretaries of the WFN Problem Commissions.

Ludo van Bogaert had decided to organize the meeting at the Institute Bunge in Antwerp in December 1964 (30, 31). The meeting was called because the financial resources of the WFN were running low.

Van Bogart thought that now was the time to create a new and separate organization, the World Association of Neurological Commissions (WANC), because that would save money for the WFN. Macdonald Critchley disagreed. He thought this was wrong, and that the research arm was essential for the WFN to survive.

Van Bogaert's plan was that decentralization included a possibility for financial support from each region. However, establishing WFN regional secretariats would have considerable costs, and outside help might be required. The plan therefore gave no support for the financial problems of the WFN. The NINDB grant terminated after 1965. The WFN would then have to become more self-sustaining with respect to administrative and programming activities. Ludo van Bogaert's presidency had been successful, but it ended in a deep financial crisis. Still, during these eight years, the organization had demonstrated its viability and prospects.

The secretaries had come together to settle the measures to be taken to enable their Problem Commissions to survive after 1965, when the NINDB grant would be terminated. Various measures were discussed, such as applying to NATO, the Warsaw Treaty, national governments, the World Health Organization (WHO), and pharmaceutical companies, but none of these was regarded likely to support the WFN. Van Bogaert then presented his idea of creating an association formed by all the Commissions, whose Executive Committee would be composed of the Secretaries. The name of the association was the World Association of Neurological Commissions (WANC). Each Commission should be able to assume its secretarial expenses. There was agreement that Adolphe Franceschetti should become the President of the WANC, and David Klein

Vice President and Secretary-Treasurer General. Franceschetti and Klein agreed provided that the WFN Executive Committee approved of the establishing of the WANC, and that the Secretaries of the Commissions, who would meet in Vienna on 4 September 1965, also confirmed the wish, expressed on 12 December 1964.

So they did. But the new structure proved to be short-lived.

Macdonald Critchley: the WFN flourishes in spite of financial problems

At the International Congress in Vienna 1965, the Council of Delegates elected Macdonald Critchley as President and Henry Miller as Secretary-Treasurer General. There were no alternative candidates.

Macdonald Critchley (1900–1997) (Fig. 2.5) was the second President of the WFN. He was born in Bristol on 2 February 1900 and matriculated from the Christian Brothers' College in Bristol at the age of 15. Since he was too young to go to university, he began to learn German to add to his considerable skills in French and Latin while waiting to be admitted to Bristol University. The following year, the First World War broke out, and by 1917 he was in the Army. In 1918, he became a cadet in the Royal Flying Corps. During this period he began to learn Russian, adding to his wide linguistic knowledge. During the Second World War, he was called upon to organize the neurological and psychiatric services for the Royal Navy. During the Second World War he was a Consulting Neurologist in the Royal Navy Volunteer Reserve based on the Royal Drake. His wartime observations in the Arctic and in the tropics provided the substance of

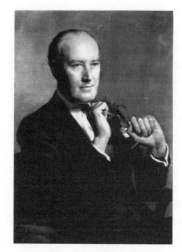

Fig. 2.5 Macdonald Critchley, the Second WFN President. WFN Flourishes in Spite of Financial Problems.

Courtesy of Lord Walton.

his Croonian lecture to the College in 1945 on the problems of naval warfare under climatic extremes. Macdonald Critchley was made Commander of the Order of the British Empire (CBE).

When the First World War was over, he returned to Bristol University and graduated at the age of 21 with first class honours. He came to London, first to Great Ormond Street, then to Maida Vale in 1923. He then arrived at Queen Square. From then on, his professional life centred on King's College Hospital and the National Hospital. He joined the house staff, which he found 'to be something like entering the Valley of the Kings at Luxor'. He felt surrounded by the ghosts of such distinguished physicians as Brown-Séquard, David Ferrier, Bastian, Beevor, Batten, William Fergusson, Marcus Gunn, Charles Balance, and Felix Semon. James Samuel Risien Russell had been on the consultant staff with John Hughlings Jackson, Sir William Gowers, Sir David Ferrier, and Sir Victor Horsley. Macdonald Critchley became the house physician of Sir Gordon Holmes, whom he felt shone brightest among the galaxy of stars surrounding him. He later became Dean of the Institute at Queen Square, and no one else accumulated such a fund of knowledge about the founders of British neurology (28–30).

At the same time, few neurologists other than Macdonald Critchley in 'The training of a neurologist' (1979) have underlined the importance of international contacts and of an acquisition of the French and German languages (35). His research interests were broad, and ranged from movement disorders and higher cerebral function to medical history. His contributions to neurology depended on his knowledge, memory, power of observation, and systematic understanding and dissection of human sensibility and behaviour. The best known of his works are those on aphasia and the parietal lobes. He was the author of over 200 published articles on neurology and 20 books, including *The Parietal Lobes*, *Aphasiology*, and the biographies of James Parkinson and Sir William Gowers.

Headache was one of his many interests. He started a Headache Clinic at King's College Hospital and was one of the founders of the 'British Migraine Trust'. He delivered a paper at the 'First Migraine Symposium' in 1966 on 'Migraine: from Cappadocia to Queen Square', combining his clinical interest with his love of history.

Macdonald Critchley knew the WFN from its formation. He had been a friend of Ludo van Bogaert, and had participated in the discussions in Brussels when the organization was conceived. He was very active in one of the most active Problem Commissions: Language Disorders (later named aphasiology).

Macdonald Critchley served as President of the Association of British Neurologists, and of the neurology section of the Royal Society of Medicine. He was the first elected Vice President of the Royal College of Physicians, and his last great public office was as president of the World Federation of Neurology (32–34).

Macdonald Critchley was one of the most intelligent and articulate neurologists of his generation, and became an outstanding leader of the organization. His Secretary-Treasurer General, Henry Miller, was a charismatic and ebullient personality. They made their mark on the meetings and congresses, and both were unanimously re-elected for a further four years at the World Congress of Neurology in 1969 (36).

The World 1965–1973: Vietnam War and the first men on the moon

The world had changed since the formation of the first WFN in 1957, but the Cold War persisted. In 1968, Soviet and Warsaw Treaty troops invaded Czechoslovakia. The Vietnam War, which ended with the fall of Saigon in 1975, influenced politics, attitudes, and personal relationships all over the world. For the USA, the years between 1961 and 1969 showed the greatest economic growth in American history. In 1969, Neil Armstrong and Edwin Aldrin became the first men to set foot on the moon. China became a member of the United Nations (UN) in 1971, and President Nixon visited the People's Republic of China in 1972. More than 30 African nations had won their independence, and the Nigerian civil war ended in 1970. The first Congress of the Pan African Association of Neurological Sciences (PAANS) was held in Cairo, Egypt, in 1973.

These years were important for the neurosciences. Neuroimaging with CT began in 1971. The Nobel Prize in Physiology or Medicine 1967 was awarded jointly to Ragnar Granit, Haldan Keffer Hartline, and George Wald for their discoveries concerning the primary physiological and chemical visual processes in the eye, and in 1970 jointly to Sir Bernard Katz, Ulf von Euler, and Julius Axelrod for their discoveries concerning the humoral transmitters in the nerve terminals and the mechanism for their storage, release, and inactivation.

Macdonald Critchley's presidency

Ludo van Bogaert was the WFN President in the critical period when the organization found its form. The economic basis of the WFN was relatively solid from the beginning because of the support from the NINDB. Macdonald Critchley took over when the structure to a great extent had been attained, but the flow of US seed money had come to an end. In his report to the Council of Delegates in New York in 1969, he stated:

> In many ways it has been a challenge, for nowadays the financial resources of the Federation are—to put it mildly—minimal. The income received each year from each of

THE SHAPING OF THE ORGANIZATION | **37**

the national societies just, only just, meets the day to day expenses entailed in an intensive world-wide correspondence. Unfortunately, it is no longer possible to meet the expenses of travel, and regrettably it is no longer feasible to give financial support to the secretariat and delegates who put in such hard work in connection with the various Research Groups, symposia, etc. (37).

In his last speech to the Council of Delegates, in Barcelona in 1973, he was even clearer:

I like to believe that I shall be leaving a flourishing and active Federation, whose prestige stands very high among neurologists throughout the world. Bonds of friendship have been cemented between our colleagues upon a truly international scale. The Federation is, I believe, a veritable United Nations of Neurology, free, however, from all racial, political, geographical, or cultural disagreements. The WFN is an organization, which is steadily growing in stature and authority, and within the past few weeks a very promising and essentially practical association has materialized between us and the World Health Organization—a bond which I hope and indeed expect will prove highly advantageous both to our Federation and to WHO.

The duties of the President have been arduous, and have entailed no little financial and working effort. However, I have never had any regrets, and am now in a position to say that the administration has been not only very exacting, but that it has been handicapped by financial stringency. An increase in subscription would go some way towards keeping pace with running costs.

If anything has been attained during the past eight years, it is due to the friendship and warmth I have received from the individual members of neurological societies literally on a worldwide scale. They have been unanimous in their generous support, and I would like here and now to express my most sincere appreciation of the help they have extended to me (34).

Ludo van Bogaert had been anxious about the WFN's future. He had described three possibilities to save the organization: an increase of the annual due from US$1 to US$2, a decentralization plan, and a new daughter organization, the WANC. None of them succeeded. The dues were not increased until at the end of Critchley's administration. No decentralization took place. The WANC had become an explosive element that almost threatened the existence of the organization.

How could the WFN then survive? Macdonald Critchley was able to see that every cloud has a silver lining. He induced a feeling of pioneer optimism in the organization. The work of the WFN not only continued, it was flourishing, in spite of a miserable economy. The orientation of the Federation remained truly international, harmonious, and stimulating.

The reason lay in the vitality of the organization. No new administrative initiatives could be taken, but the activity that had been induced in the Research Groups was high. During Macdonald Critchley's presidency, a new Research Group, on Extrapyramidal Disease, held its first business meeting in 1972, organized by Dr Melvin Yahr. Three other and very active Research Groups had been formed, the Research Group on Motor Neuron Disease, the Research Group on Industrial and Environmental Neurology (later renamed Environmental Neurology), and the Research Group on Neuropaediatrics. But they were now Research Groups, not Problem Commissions. What had happened to the WANC?

WFN Executive Committee meeting 4 September 1965

Forty-two delegates and/or authorized representatives of member societies of the WFN convened for the WFN Executive Committee meeting held on 4 September 1965 in the Palais Palffy, Vienna. The President, Ludo van Bogaert was ill and could not attend. Therefore Pearce Bailey chaired the meeting. The WFN Executive Committee approved unanimously the proposal for the formation of the WANC. Critchley urged the delegates of all societies who were delinquent with the annual member society dues to bring their accounts up to date. It was also decided that no change be made in the present Constitution or organization of the WFN—that is, no decentralization. Macdonald Critchley was then elected new President of the WFN, while van Bogaert was given the title of Président Fondateur, and Pearce Bailey that of Honorary Secretary-General (39).

The WANC war: a meeting in Geneva

During the first years of its existence, the economy of the WFN had been based upon generous support from the NINDB. From 1965, it was clear that no further funding for WFN activities would come from US Government sources. The hope was that the WFN now would be able to generate its own income.

Ludo van Bogaert had proposed in 1964 to include all Problem Commissions in the new organization called the World Association of Neurological Commissions (WANC). He had hoped that WANC should be able to raise sufficient funds. Klaus Zülch (chairman of the Commission on Neuro-Oncology), Ernst Frauchiger, and Adolphe Franceschetti supported van Bogaert's proposal, but several colleagues had strong objections. The WFN Executive Committee approved the proposal.

However, strong antagonism to the idea of a new and partly rival organization appeared. Its relationship to WFN was unclear, and it seemed to be informally and only loosely associated with the WFN. In spite of the economic constraints, meetings of the Problem Commissions had been held through support and hospitality from universities, research foundations, and drug companies and to a great extent also personal expenditure to meet the costs of travel and accommodation.

THE SHAPING OF THE ORGANIZATION | **39**

When Macdonald Critchley took over as the new WFN President, he immediately consulted the national delegates about problem with the WANC. His view was that a Federation without the research arm would be impotent. It was therefore decided that the past and present officers of the WFN with Chairmen and Secretaries of the Problem Commissions should meet in Geneva in July 1966.

Why did the meeting take place at the Institute of Ophthalmology in Geneva? Geneva is of course central in Europe, and is the home of the WHO. But more important was that Professor Adolphe Franceschetti was based there, and had held the Chair of Ophthalmology since 1933. The eye clinic was one of the most impressive in the world, and Franceschetti had a high international standing in neuro-ophthalmology. In 1945, he had founded a genetics department at his eye clinic, entrusted to Dr David Klein. Franceschetti was elected President of the new organization, the WANC.

The atmosphere at the Geneva meeting was ideal. According to John Walton, 'The quality of food and drink provided in the warm surroundings of the Institute of Ophthalmology was such that even Henry Miller approved. Hence, by the time that the meeting began the spirit of confrontation which had seemed likely had been slightly tempered' (36).

The discussion was indeed difficult, with van Bogaert and Critchley as the two opponents. John Walton suggested as a compromise that the WFN should create a Research Committee with its own Chairman and Secretary-Treasurer General, who should be accepted as officers of the Federation but would remain under the authority of the President and the Secretary-Treasurer General of the WFN as a whole. The proposal was accepted, and van Bogaert, Critchley and Miller were able to shake hands. The WFN Executive Committee (later renamed the Council of Delegates) supported the dissolution of the WANC. The WFN Research Committee was born. By this compromise, John Walton had saved the organization from collapse.

The differences of opinion had been dramatic, and John Walton's proposal was to create a new organizational unit of the WFN, the Research Committee. The Problem Commissions were now renamed 'Research Groups' and organized in the new Research Committee. The Secretaries of these Research Groups would form the Research Committee, as before. Elected as the President and the Secretary-Treasurer General of the Research Committee were those who had been candidates for the corresponding offices of the original WANC, Adolphe Franceschetti and his close friend, David Klein of the Institute of Medical Genetics in Geneva. Franceschetti died in 1968, and it was unanimously decided that Professor Ernst Frauchiger of Bern should succeed him as Chairman of the Research Committee.

The hope was that each Research Group would bring money to the organization. A few did, but many Research Groups were unable to support the WFN financially. John Walton's idea was that some Problem Commissions— now Research Groups—might develop into international societies that could become corporate members of the Research Committee with the payment of an annual subscription which might improve the economy of the organization. This proved to be a great step forward. But it took several years until it worked. In the meantime, the economic situation of the WFN remained critical.

By 1969, the income of the Research Committee was only sufficient to support the secretarial and administrative expenses of the Committee. No grants were available to the Research Groups to support their activities. (40)

The Research Committee: oil upon troubled water

It was made clear in the minutes from the Geneva meeting, 1–2 July 1966, that the Executive Committee (Council of Delegates) of the WFN intended to reverse their actions taken in Vienna, as they had not then appreciated all the implications. After considerable discussion, a resolution dissolving the WANC and establishing in its place the Research Committee of the WFN was agreed by the meeting.

The Executive Committee met at the Neurological Institute, New York on 25 June 1967. In the period following the Geneva and Vienna meetings, there had been continued discussions about the WANC and the Research Committee. It was the term 'dissolving' that now created problems.

The prize of the peace was a proclamation drawn up as coming from the President of the WFN to be read aloud at this Executive Committee meeting. The new Secretary-Treasurer General, Henry Miller, read out the document:

> The Council of the Research Committee of the World Federation of Neurology, at its meeting in Geneva on 27th May, again expressed regret concerning the misunderstandings which had arisen between the Executive Committee of the World Association of Neurological Commissions (WANC) on the one hand and the President of the World Federation of Neurology on the other. They re-affirmed that the WANC was never intended to be a rival organization to the WFN but that it was always proposed, following its foundation meeting in Antwerp in 1964 that the WANC would operate wholly within the framework of the WFN. They wish to point out that the statement in the Report of the President of the WFN for 1966 that the WANC had now been dissolved was in their opinion incorrect, but that according to the agreed Resolution passed in Geneva on 2nd July 1966 the organization was reconstituted as the Research Committee of the WFN.
>
> The President of the WFN also expressed regret if he had misinterpreted in his letter to the delegates and Annual Report the spirit and intention of the original formation of the WANC. It was agreed that following unanimous approval by the Council of its

new Statutes, the Research Committee of the WFN intended in the future to work harmoniously together to further the cause of world-wide research in the neurological sciences (41).

There was no discussion.

Collaboration with other disciplines

A symposium with neurosurgery led to a successful symposium on the Late Effects of Head Injuries in Washington in 1969 and was attended by over 2000. The World Psychiatric Association and the WFN also sponsored a symposium on dementia in London in 1970.

The Research Group on Neurochemistry was disbanded after an International Society of Neurochemistry had been established. That society had in many ways developed from the Research Group established by the World Federation.

WFN and WHO

The association between the WHO and the WFN was established during Macdonald Critchley's presidency. The WHO had constituted a small, but distinguished, ad hoc committee to consider the special problems of tropical neurology. It was hoped that important developments might emerge in which the Research Groups on Tropical Neurology would play a role.

New York 1969

The World Congress of Neurology took place in New York in 1969. Macdonald Critchley and Henry Miller were unanimously re-elected WFN President and Secretary-Treasurer General.

The activity of the Research Groups

The Research Group on Neuromuscular Disorders, under the leadership of Professor John Walton, soon became one of the largest and most productive. Their first international congress took place in Perth, Australia, in 1971, followed by a second in Newcastle-upon-Tyne, UK, in 1974.

The Research Group on Extrapyramidal Disease gradually developed into an international organization with corporate membership of the Research Committee. The Research Group on Huntington's chorea had a highly successful symposium under the leadership of Professor André Barbeau, in Columbus, Ohio, in 1972 to honour the centenary of the publication of George Huntington's classical paper. The Research Group on Headache and Migraine met in London in 1972, and in Barcelona in 1973. Several of the Research Groups met during these years, exchanged information, and inspired to research.

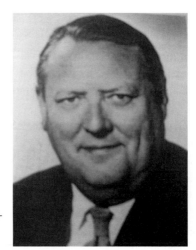

Fig. 2.6 Henry Miller (1913–1976) Secretary-General of the Federation of World Neurology.

Journal of Neurological Sciences 1976, 30:423–425. Copyright Elsevier.

Neurology in Africa

During Macdonald Critchley's presidency, there was an important upsurge of interest in the neurological sciences on the African continent. There had been an African symposium on neurology in 1966, and another in Ibadan, Nigeria, in 1970. A lack of definite and reliable information on the pattern of neurological diseases on the African continent soon became visible.

The WFN Research Group on Tropical and Geographical Neurology met in Lagos, Nigeria, in 1971. There was an agreement that the definition of the disease pattern in different parts of Africa should start with tumours of the nervous system. Professor Renato Ruberti of Kenya organized a symposium for this purpose in Nairobi, Kenya, in 1972. The Pan African Association of Neurological Sciences (PAANS) was founded there, and an impressive first meeting of PAANS was held in Cairo, Egypt, in April 1973 (42).

Henry Miller (1913–1976) Secretary-General Treasurer, World Federation of Neurology, 1965–1973

Henry Miller (Fig. 2.6) was the WFN Secretary-Treasurer General during Macdonald Critchley's presidency. He died suddenly and unexpectedly in 1976.

Born in Stockton-on-Tees in December 1913, Henry Miller was a dedicated north-easterner throughout his life and was one of the most distinguished graduates of the Newcastle-upon-Tyne College of Medicine at the University of Durham. After house officer posts in Newcastle and a period of training in pathology at the Johns Hopkins Hospital in Baltimore and following a brief flirtation with paediatrics under the influence of the late Sir James Spence, who was inevitably attracted by his energy, high intelligence, and ebullient personality, he embarked

THE SHAPING OF THE ORGANIZATION | 43

upon a career in clinical medicine and neurology on the advice of Professor F. J. Natrass. During his service as a neuropsychiatrist in the RAF, a period of fruitful training and experience in which he was greatly influenced by Sir Charles Symonds, having already acquired the MD and MRCP, he went on to acquire a Diploma in Psychological Medicine, a qualification which after many verbal brushes with colleagues in psychological medicine, he subsequently suppressed, even though he had a deep interest in psychiatry which he regarded as 'neurology without physical signs'. After demobilization he underwent further training at Hammersmith and at the National Hospital, Queen Square, before being appointed Assistant Physician to the Royal Victoria Infirmary, Newcastle-upon-Tyne, in 1947. Following this return to his beloved north-east, new distinctions followed rapidly. For several years he prospered as a busy and much sought after consultant in part-time private practice. His forthright handling of some difficult patients occasionally caused offence but more often proved almost miraculously effective. Generations of medical students and house staff owe much to his inspired teaching and example, and even senior colleagues never ceased to marvel that, being so quick, he was nevertheless so often right. Later he established a new department of neurology, firmly based in both clinical work and research, which grew rapidly and acquired an international reputation. His own research on multiple sclerosis, on accident neurosis and on many diverse neurological topics won him wide renown and his review articles, many published in the *British Medical Journal*, were widely read and quoted, as were his outspoken criticisms of deficiencies in the National Health Service. He was appointed to a personal chair of neurology in 1964, became Dean of Medicine in 1966 and Vice-Chancellor of the University of Newcastle-upon-Tyne in 1968, an appointment that he occupied at the moment of his untimely death.

How can one possibly find words to do justice to this remarkable man? His energy, his drive, his remarkable intuitive clinical ability, his abounding flow of language, spiked with barbs of (at times) slightly wounding wit, but above all his limitless generosity to friends, colleagues, and junior staff were extraordinary. Books could be (and probably will be) filled with quotations from his tongue and from his fertile pen, some few of which were hallowed for posterity as 'Henry Millerisms' in a popular medical journal. Who can forget such comments as, 'The best instrument for obtaining the plantar response is the ignition key of a Bentley', or, 'Hemiplegic multiple sclerosis is a rarity and is to be diagnosed only by me'. And there are many more such which we shall all remember with sadness but with gratitude. If not always popular with his peers, who frequently misunderstood (and more often misinterpreted) his roguish wit, he was loved and respected by his juniors and contemporaries, especially by those who worked closely with and knew him best and readily forgave his at times outrageous but impish comments; above all, he will be mourned by his students whose adulation came little short of worship. Foreign and national honours were showered upon him: visiting professor in many universities overseas, honorary member of many national neurological associations, Secretary-General of the WFN, Chairman of the BMA Planning Unit, President of the Association of Physicians of Great Britain and Ireland; these and many more distinctions came his way. His years of office in the WFN, during Dr Macdonald Critchley's presidency, brought his conspicuous talents to the attention of a worldwide audience of neurologists to whom he was invariably an impressive figure; and when he was there, the meetings were never dull. Clinical neurology was his first love, writing his second, not only will his textbooks and scientific papers be a lasting memorial to this man of stature, but also so will his perspicacious monograph on *Medicine and Society* and his wickedly provocative but thoughtful articles in *The Listener*. Always a bon viveur and lover of the arts, a man of wide culture despite his outward buffoonery, he strode through life with an aura owing something to Max Beerbohm and perhaps also to Rabelais.

When the new Newcastle undergraduate medical curriculum was introduced in 1962, Henry was one of its most outspoken critics and was heard to say 'Curriculum review is an occupational disease of Deans which simply results in the same subjects being taught in a different order.' But when he himself became Dean he also became a firm convert to the new order and one of its staunchest advocates. He had many critics, especially among those who were the recipients of his verbal onslaughts, but he loved a spirited riposte and was never reluctant to admit either that he was wrong or that he had been bested in an argument. As Vice-Chancellor his skill in handling the student body was matchless and all will agree that there never was or will be another Vice-Chancellor like Henry. With senior academics, students, porters, clerks, or visitors, however distinguished, he was superbly unpredictable, original, and always irreverently cheerful. Medicine, neurology, and the academic world will be much poorer for his passing; if the reader will forgive the cliché, as he certainly would not, he was an unforgettable character. He will be remembered not as a copy of some or several great men of yesteryear but as the one and only Henry Miller. He is survived by his loyal, charming and vigorous wife, Eileen, and two sons and two daughters; we would wish them to know that it was a privilege to have known and worked with him.

Sigvald Refsum: the WFN defining its position

At the World Congress of Neurology in Barcelona in 1973, Sigvald Refsum (1907–1991) (Fig. 2.7) was unanimously elected President of the WFN. There were no alternative candidates. He chose as his Secretary-Treasurer General,

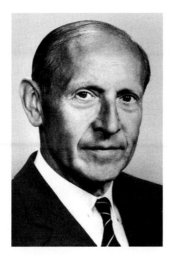

Fig. 2.7 Sigvald Refsum, the Third WFN President. WFN defining its position.
The archives of the WFN.

Professor Bent de Fine Olivarius of Aarhus, Denmark (1922–2005). It turned out, however, that Olivarius had severe health problems, and Professor Palle Juul-Jensen, also of Aarhus, had to take over in 1977 due to Dr Olivarius' illness.

The first WFN President, Ludo van Bogaert, had managed to establish the new organization. During the presidency of Macdonald Critchley, van Bogaert's successor, there still was a feeling of pioneer optimism in the organization and the federation was flourishing, in spite of a miserable economy. It was now up to the new administration to define its position and responsibilities.

Sigvald Bernhard Refsum was born in Gransherad, Norway, on 8 May 1907, the son of Sigvald Refsum, a church minister. He graduated in medicine from Rikshospitalet, Oslo, in 1932. Refsum trained in psychiatry and in neurology, starting his career in 1936 under Professor Georg H. Monrad-Krohn at the Department of Neurology, the National Hospital (Rikshospitalet) Oslo.

Refsum soon became interested in a family in which several members suffered from a neurological condition that had not been described previously, characterized by cerebellar ataxia, polyneuropathy, and atypical retinitis pigmentosa. Nerve deafness and electrocardiographic changes are common but inconsistent features. He called it *heredopathia atactica polyneuritiformis*, now better known as Refsum's disease. This was the subject for his PhD thesis, which he defended in 1946. In 1963, it was discovered that patients with Refsum's disease, which is potentially lethal, had an accumulation of phytanic acid, and the biochemical defect was shown in 1967 to be a deficiency in its α-oxidation.

Refsum spent several years in academic centres in the USA. He was visiting professor at the Illinois University, Chicago, 1949–1950, at the University of Minnesota in Minneapolis 1950–1951 and then at the University of

California in San Francisco 1951–1952. Sigvald Refsum published more than 120 scientific papers.

In 1952, he was appointed the first professor of neurology at the University of Bergen, the second medical school to be established in Norway. In 1954, he succeeded Monrad-Krohn as professor of neurology at the University of Oslo, a position which he held until he retired in 1978.

Refsum was a shy and self-effacing man, kind, and judicious and a statesman-like neurologist. His quietly firm and effective leadership soon won for him a place in the regard and affection of his countrymen (43,44).

The world 1973–1981: political tension and oil embargo

The Vietnam War ended in 1975. The US economy strained under the pressure of the OPEC-imposed oil embargo of 1973. The Soviet Union was at the peak of its power in the early 1970s, but its vigorous economy fell victim to central planning and raw materials allocation.

The Soviet army invaded Afghanistan in 1979 and withdrew in 1989. Ayatollah Khomeini (1902–1989) was a leader of the Iranian Revolution and came to power in Iran in 1979. Ronald Reagan (1911–2004) was elected US President in 1980, and took office in 1981, following Jimmy Carter, who had been elected in 1976. Margaret Thatcher became Britain's first female Prime Minister in 1979.

The Nobel Prize in Physiology or Medicine 1976 was awarded jointly to Baruch S. Blumberg and D. Carleton Gajdusek for their discoveries concerning new mechanisms for the origin and dissemination of infectious diseases, with focus upon the pathogenesis of kuru and Creutzfeldt–Jacob diseases. In 1979, the Nobel Prize in Physiology or Medicine was awarded jointly to Allan M. Cormack and Godfrey N. Hounsfield for the development of computer-assisted tomography. This opened a new era in diagnostics in neurology. The Nobel Prize in Physiology or Medicine 1980 was awarded jointly to Baruj Benacerraf, Jean Dausset, and George D. Snell for their discoveries concerning genetically determined structures on the cell surface that regulate immunological reactions. Their findings have considerable consequences for the understanding of important neurological conditions such as multiple sclerosis.

Refsum's presidency

Refsum had to face a series of economic and constitutional problems when he took over as WFN President in 1973. The financial support from NINDB, which had been crucial for WFN during its first years, was now part of history (45). The main income would be the annual dues, which more or less ceased to exist. Refsum even had problems in reimbursing his own WFN travels. There were therefore few new activities of the WFN organization, and Refsum's

THE SHAPING OF THE ORGANIZATION | **47**

prime function had to be the representation of WFN at international meetings, which he performed with style and dignity.

In spite of a severe financial crisis, the activity of some of the Federation's Research Groups was impressive. The Research Group on Neuromuscular Diseases had had over 1000 participants at their successful congress in Montreal in 1978. There was a great upsurge of interest in Parkinsonism in the late 1960s with new research data on the role of dopamine deficiency in the pathogenesis of Parkinson's disease. Professor Melvin Yahr had organized the first Research Group on Extrapyramidal Disease, which rapidly monitored the development in treatment of this disease (46). The new Research Group on Neurotoxicology had held its first symposium, the proceedings of which were published by Raven Press. André Barbeau of Montreal had formed a new Research Group on heredoataxias. It had been agreed with the International Society for Pediatric Neurology that that society would be represented on the WFN Research Committee.

The new WFN journal, the *Journal of the Neurological Sciences* with John Walton as Editor-in-Chief, made significant progress, and in 1974 for the first time the Elsevier Publishing Company found it possible to make a financial contribution towards the cost of defraying editorial and other expenses (47). After being Editor-in-Chief of the Journal for 11 years, and now appointed Chairman of the Research Committee, John Walton decided that the time had come for a change, and Professor Walter Bryan Matthews of Oxford (1920–2001) became his successor as the new Editor-in-Chief (47).

In 1977, John Walton was appointed Chairman of the Research Committee. He had been instrumental in its development, and reviewed and revised its constitution. From now on, the WFN Research Committee became the pivot of the Research Group activities of the Federation. A Newsletter of the Research Committee followed, which contained an up-to-date list of the Research Groups and of their officers (48)

The second WFN financial crisis

The second financial crisis occurred during Refsum's presidency. Unfortunately, Olivarius, the Secretary-Treasurer General, had not written to the national societies to remind them of the annual dues, and for about one year no money was brought into the organization. Transfer of money from England to Denmark after the new administration had taken over was complicated, and the WFN funds of £8000 were transferred in June 1974 (45).

At the Council of Delegates in Amsterdam, 1975, Secretary-Treasurer General Olivarius reported to the national delegates:

Times have changed in the WFN. I remember the first glorious years, when financial means were nearly unlimited, as it seemed, thanks to the subsidy from the United States Government—a period when newly elected member societies were presented with gilt-edged certificates of membership . . .

Since the American subsidy was withdrawn the WFN has been left to support itself on the dues received from member-societies, and you all know that this has not been enough to initiate expansion in the activities of the WFN—especially as many member countries never pay their dues. . . .

May I add that the costs of administration have never been as low in the history of the WFN? There have been no expenses for offices or secretarial assistance, which is carried out within the hospital working hours, and the postage and telephone calls have been paid by our hospitals or personally by the officers (46).

In 1977, Professor Palle Juul-Jensen (Aarhus, Denmark) was appointed Assistant Secretary, according to the constitution of the WFN. His appointment required ratification by the members of the Council, and Juul-Jensen was elected Acting Secretary-Treasurer General after Olivarius, and he remained in office during Refsum's presidency.

The financial situation of the WFN was weak during the first part of Refsum's administration. Although the costs of administration had never been so low, the income was minimal, and the Secretary-Treasurer was unable to present an audited balance at the meeting of the Council of Delegates in 1975 (46). It improved under the able leadership of Palle Juul-Jensen, who took over under very difficult circumstances, but the cost of administration, including travel expenses, had to be kept low (47).

Amsterdam 1977

The World Congress of Neurology in 1977 took place in Amsterdam. Sigvald Refsum was re-elected WFN President. John Walton was appointed Chairman of the Research Committee. It was agreed that all national societies affiliated to the organization should be asked to pay a subscription equivalent to US$2.00 per member each year to the WFN in support of its activities.

Professor George Bruyn, who was the Secretary of the Amsterdam congress, was elected chairman of the new WFN Finance Committee. The Finance Committee, and later also the Council of Delegates, decided that subscriptions from individual members of research groups collected centrally by the Treasurer of the Research Committee should be discontinued, and that the research groups should raise funds for the support of their groups, of which 10% would be paid to WFN central funds for administrative costs of the Research Committee (48).

The development of the WFN Research Committee

The new Chairman of the Research Committee, John Walton, consulted with the existing research groups. It had already become clear that activities originally initiated by some WFN Research Groups had ultimately developed into international societies. It was now decided that in future their Secretaries, alongside representatives of the Research Groups, where appropriate, might represent such international societies, on the Research Committee. One example is the Research Group on Neurochemistry, which was dissolved in 1978. From then on, the International Society of Neurochemistry would represent this discipline upon the Research Committee in the person of its Secretary.

In other instances it might become appropriate for the research groups to be disbanded if their role in promoting international collaboration in research in the discipline concerned had been assumed by the international society.

The Research Group on Pediatric Neurology is another example. In consultation with the International Society for Pediatric Neurology, it was agreed that its Secretary-General would represent that Society on the Research Committee.

A meeting of the WFN Research Committee in Newcastle-upon-Tyne on 30 March 1979 followed the Newsletter of the Research Committee, and the Statutes of the Research Committee were published (50, 51).

The role of the WFN Research Committee in the future

Organization of World Congresses of Neurology

At the meeting of the Research Committee in Amsterdam 1977, it was agreed that one of its future roles should be to put before the Organizing Committee of future International Congresses of Neurology themes which they wanted the Committee to consider for possible inclusion in the programme. Professor van Bogaert had suggested this as early as 1957.

It was on this basis that the Research Committee proposed topics that would be central at the upcoming World Congress of Neurology in Kyoto in 1981 (52).

The WFN Research Group on Cerebrovascular Disease

In 1979 the Research Group on Cerebral Sirkulasjon became the Research Group on Cerebrovascular Disease. Professor Klaus Zülch retired from being Secretary of the Group in 1979. David Klein was the Research Committee Secretary Treasurer, and $10,665.65 was transferred to the WFN in 1987.

A major activity of the group was that of sponsoring the biennial Salzburg Conference on Cerebral Vascular Disease. It was first agreed that all 400 individuals registered with that conference should be invited to become members of the Research Group. It was involved in organizing international symposia, and gradually its activities became so central to neurosciences that international stroke organizations have developed. Helmut Lechner, Carlo Loeb, John Marshall, and John Stirling Meyer would now form the Executive Committee of the Research Group in addition to the original charter members of the Salzburg conference. In 1979, it was decided that, from now on, the Research Group on Cerebral Vascular Disease of the WFN should organize the Salzburg Conference only (49).

The Salzburg Conference group gradually became stagnant with very little involvement of active researchers. The Research Group on Cerebrovascular Diseases and its main activity, the Salzburg Conference, therefore became less relevant. The advances in stroke were now first reported at the International Stroke Conference of the American Heart Association, and later at the European Stroke Conference too. It was actually the Japanese who began an International Stroke Society (ISS), holding the first World Stroke Congress in 1989 in Kyoto.

Subsequently, James Toole founded the World Stroke Federation (WSF), and Antonio Culebras became President. In 2004, Julien Bogousslavsky became President of the ISS. It was obvious that the world did not need two international stroke organizations. They began acting as one, with dual officers but one President. It culminated in the legal integration of the ISS/WSF, and during the World Stroke Congress held in Cape Town in October 2006 it became (after a vote) the World Stroke Organization.

WFN and WHO

The Federation's relations with the WHO had expanded, and the WFN now had the status of a non-governmental organization affiliated to the WHO. The association between the WFN and the WHO, which was established during Macdonald Critchley's presidency, continued to develop, and a section of Neurosciences was formed in connection with the office of Mental Health of the WHO with Professor Diana Bolis as section leader. It became clear, however, that that organization did not draw upon internationally recognized expertise in their field, and the collaboration of the two organizations was therefore not optimal.

Refsum participated in the WHO Consultation on Neurosciences, but the WHO found that the activities of the WFN were slow—to a great extent based upon the poor financial situation of the WFN.

Richard Masland: progress in the organization of the WFN

At the meeting of the Council of Delegates of the World Federation of Neurology held during the 12th World Congress of Neurology in Kyoto, Japan, in 1981, Richard Masland (Fig. 2.8) was elected WFN President and Sir John Walton First Vice President. Pierre Dreyfus (USA) was elected Secretary-Treasurer General with Palle Juul-Jensen (Denmark) Joint Secretary-Treasurer General.

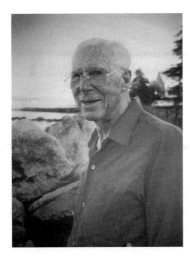

Fig. 2.8 Richard Masland, the Fourth WFN President. Progress in the organization of the WFN.

The archives of the WFN.

Mahmoud Mustafa (Egypt), Endre Csanda (Hungary), Carlo Loeb (Italy), Antonio Spina-Franca (Brazil), and Shibanosuke Katsuki (Japan) were elected Vice Presidents, and Walter Bryan Matthews continued as Editor-in-Chief of the *Journal of the Neurological Sciences*. In 1983, George Bruyn was appointed the new Editor-in-Chief after Bryan Matthews.

Richard Lambert Masland (1910–2003) was born in Philadelphia, USA. He attended Haverford College and the University of Pennsylvania School of Medicine. Masland received his medical degree from the University of Pennsylvania School of Medicine in 1935. After an internship at the Pennsylvania Hospital and a fellowship in neurology at the Hospital of the University of Pennsylvania, he became an associate in neurology in 1940. Thereafter, he served from 1942 to 1945 as director of the department of physiology at the US Army School of Aviation Medicine.

Richard Masland became professor of neurology and psychiatry at the Bowman Gray School of Medicine at Wake Forest College in Winston-Salem, North Carolina, 1952–1957, during which time he was also research director of the National Association for Retarded Children.

From 1959 to 1968 he succeeded Pearce Bailey as the director of the NINDB. He is known for leading the National Collaborative Perinatal Project, a nationwide study of pregnancy and child development, between 1959 and 1966. The study followed more than 50 000 women from the time of their pregnancies until their children reached the age of eight. He then became chair of the Department of Neurology at the College of Physicians and Surgeons of Columbia University in New York. In 1973, he became H. Houston Merritt Professor of Neurology, emeritus. He was the president of the American Epilepsy Society and the New York Neurological Society (53).

Masland was unanimously elected as President of the World Federation of Neurology, and was highly appreciated for his judgment, scientific credibility, and clinical expertise. He apparently ran his office on a shoestring from his own home and with minimal secretarial support, but was extremely effective and hard working (36).

The world 1981–1989: perestroika, Chernobyl and the Berlin Wall

Mikhail Gorbachev, the leader of the Soviet Union, initiated his new policy of perestroika and its radical reforms. In 1988, he also introduced *glasnost*, which gave new freedom to the Soviet people, including freedom of speech. In 1986, during the annual meeting of the American Academy of Neurology in New Orleans, a nuclear reactor at Chernobyl exploded and clouds of radioactive isotopes spread over much of Europe. In October 1981, President Anwar El Sadat of Egypt was assassinated and Hosny Mubarak became his successor. The brief but undeclared war between Argentina and Great Britain over control of the Falklands Islands discredited Argentina's military government and helped lead to the restoration of civilian rule in 1983. The Berlin Wall was torn down in 1989.

In 1981, the Nobel Prize in Physiology or Medicine was divided, one half awarded to Roger W. Sperry for his discoveries concerning the functional specialization of the cerebral hemispheres. The other half went jointly to David H. Hubel and Torsten N. Wiesel for their discoveries concerning information processing in the visual system.

In 1986, the Nobel Prize in Physiology or Medicine was divided between Stanley Cohen and Rita Levi-Montalcini for their discovery that nerve cells release growth factors that stimulate and regulate the development of the complex nervous system.

Richard Masland's presidency

Richard Masland first nominated Pierre Dreyfus as his Secretary-Treasurer General. For personal reasons, Pierre Dreyfus decided not to take up the appointment. Professor James F. Toole of Winston-Salem was then appointed and became Masland's Secretary-Treasurer General for the whole presidential period. John Walton was Chairman of the Research Committee.

One of Masland's first acts as President was a modification of the Constitution and bye-laws. The Chairman of the Research Committee should automatically become First Vice President. The Council of Delegates accepted the proposal, and John Walton became First Vice President of the WFN. Armand Lowenthal was joint (adjunct) Secretary-Treasurer General and Secretary of the Research Committee (54).

Retrospectively, these were the main challenges, which Masland met when he took over from Refsum in 1981:

1 A closer relationship between the WFN and the Research Committee was needed.

2 The relationship between the WFN and the WHO had to be improved.

3 The WFN needed a sound financial basis.

4 The use of *World Neurology* to improve the information to neurologists throughout the world.

5 Improve the quality of care for people with neurological diseases.

Of these, the main challenge was to secure the financial basis for the organization, while the one that would bring the WFN its special trademark for the future was the newsletter *World Neurology*.

Hamburg 1985

The successful World Congress of Neurology took place in Hamburg, Germany, in 1985. The new newsletter of the WFN, *World Neurology*, now appeared for the first time. At the meeting of the Council of Delegates, Richard L. Masland was re-elected WFN President, Sir John Walton First Vice President and Secretary of the Research Committee, and James F. Toole Secretary-Treasurer General. Armand Lowenthal was elected Adjunct Secretary-Treasurer General. Five Vice Presidents were elected: Ernesto Herskovits, Jose Manuel Martinez-Lage, Hirotaro Narabayashi, Shaul Feldman, and Irena Hausmanowa-Petrusewicz.

The financial situation of the WFN

The financial crisis, which had followed the Federation during the two last administrations, had become more serious, because some countries had not paid their membership fees for several years and others had paid only sporadically. The cash balance at 20 July 1981 was DKr. 134,765 equivalent to US$17,732. A circular message was sent to all national delegates drawing their attention to the provisions of the statutes and bye-laws of the Federation relating to the payment of subscriptions (52). The total income over 1983 plus the balance over 1982 amounted to US$23,679.

WFN bankrupt at the close of 1987

According to the constitution, the Council of Delegates and the WFN Standing Committees should meet at the conference centre in the year between the world congresses. The 1989 congress was to take place in New Delhi. The WFN Finance Committee therefore met in New Delhi in September 1987, before the Council of Delegates.

The economy of the WFN had brought George Bruyn, the Chairman of the committee, in sombre mood. The WFN 1986 budget was considered and approved, but the WFN budget proposed for 1987 presented serious problems.

The expenses included a proposed transfer of US$15,000 from the WFN to the host society of the country responsible for the next World Congress. If the Finance Committee accepted the proposed budget, this would exceed the income. The Finance Committee therefore had to reduce the proposed transfer to US$12,500. This was the sum that should be transferred to the 13th World Congress of Neurology as an interest-free loan (56, 57). As a result of the loan transfer, and the travel costs to be defrayed for WFN officers meeting in New Delhi on 26–28 September, and increased demands made upon the WFN, the proposed 1987 budget closed with a deficit of approximately $40,000.

This meant that the WFN would be bankrupt by the close of 1987. It was clear, Bruyn pointed out, that drastic measures could no longer be avoided. He urgently recommended the institution of an ad hoc Rescue Committee, to be discharged automatically as soon as the WFN had reached the state of solvency again.

How did WFN manage the financial crisis?

The advice of the WFN Finance Committee

On behalf of the WFN Finance Committee (WFN-FC), George Bruyn proposed to the Steering Committee and to the Council of Delegates:

a To instruct the WFN-accountants to audit all financial statements of WFN including those of all its Research Groups, from 1 January 1987.

b To urge 20 national societies who were delinquent in paying their dues over 1987, or 1986 and 1987, to pay before 1 November 1987.

c To have the WFN-accountants shift from a cash to an accrual method of accounting commencing 1 January 1987.

d Any further increase in the number of WFN-officers, which would progressively jeopardize WFN's finances, should be strongly discouraged.

e The WFN-FC recommended that a Fund-Raising Subcommittee of the WFN-FC be formed, chaired by Professor Helmut Lechner to investigate means of attracting financial support from additional sources.

f That a Publications Subcommittee of WFN-FC be formed and chaired by Professor Robert Daroff, to be charged with development of resources from WFN-sponsored journals, starting with scrutinizing the contracts of the *Journal of the Neurological Sciences*, *Journal of Neuroimmunology*, *Acta Neuropathologica* and the WFN-*World Neurology* newsletter.

g The WFN-FC considered that the annual dues for individual WFN-membership had remained unchanged at $2 for 20 years despite inflation. It recommended these dues to be raised to $5 on the basis of the following arguments:

– The WFN's state of bankruptcy,

– The steady increase of demands upon WFN,

– The analysis of the WFN-dues roster of the various national neurological societies, which showed that the brunt of such a dues-increase would be borne by 6 or 7 affluent developed countries. Dues roster: only 45% of members pay (58).

The WFN-FC, for the same purpose, recommended that the annual subsidy to *Acta Neuropathologica* be discontinued from 1 January 1988. The final agreement with Elsevier concerning the *Journal of the Neurological Sciences* had been agreed and signed. The contract with Raven Press concerning *World Neurology* was terminated on 31 December 1988, but efforts to obtain another publisher continued.

The WFN Steering Committee proposed that the Finance Committee's suggestions become effective immediately (59). The Council of Delegates convened next afternoon. The recommendation of the Finance Committee for an ad hoc committee to consider fund raising and 'rescue' from the current impecunious state was approved. The increase in membership dues to $5.00 for each member of the member associations was accepted unanimously (60).

The economy of the organization was apparently saved. The funds of the WFN treasury had now been built up from US$9,645 in 1982 to $225,000 in 1989 (61).

Masland and the Research Groups

Masland worked to obtain a closer relationship between the WFN and the WFN Research Committee. Together with John Walton, the Chairman of the Research Committee and now First Vice President, he monitored the activity of the established Research Groups as well as new fields of research that might serve as nuclei of new Research Groups.

The WFN Research Groups continued to be highly activity, and sponsored over 25 workshops, conferences, and symposia during the first part of Masland's administration. The International League against Epilepsy was established well in advance of the WFN, but there was no WFN Research Group on

Epilepsy. Masland pointed out at the beginning of his presidency the need for better contact between the two organizations. He had extensive discussions with the International League Against Epilepsy and with Epilepsy International, and it was concluded that Epilepsy International should have corporate membership of the Research Committee and be represented on the Research Committee.

A new Research Group was established for neuroimmunology. Sponsorship had been discussed for the new journal, *Journal of Neuroimmunology*, but the publisher did not regard it as being sponsored by the WFN. The WFN also participated in the First International Congress of Neuroimmunology in 1982, co-sponsored with the Istituto di Recerche Farmacologiche Mario Negri.

A new Research Group on Aging and Dementia was established in 1984, with Robert Katzman, USA, and Bernard Tomlinson, Great Britain, as co-secretaries.

A Research Group on Behavioural Neurology appeared, and it also became a corporate member of the Research Committee. Sidney Walker III (La Jolla) was the first President.

Neurological education

Masland also stressed the educational and the administrative role of the WFN. During Masland's presidency, Professor van der Lugt of the Netherlands proposed the formation of a new Research Group for Neurological Education. In the years to come, this became an important issue for the WFN administration. A fact-finding survey was suggested to determine what a neurologist is, or should be. Over time, Continuous Education became a topic for a Standing Committee more than a Research Group.

The WFN and international organizations

The WHO has the responsibility for the International Classification of Diseases (ICD). In 1982, the WHO consulted the WFN about the revision of the neurological part of the ICD and of the International Nomenclature of Disease. The WFN objected to the inclusion of cerebrovascular diseases in the cardiovascular chapter rather than in the neurological one. WFN did not succeed for the ICD-10, but considering the development of research and treatment of cerebrovascular disorders, the situation may be different in coming revisions.

In 1987, John Walton, James Toole, and Andre Lowenthal met with Dr Norman Sartorius, who was the Director of the WHO Division of Mental Health.

Richard Masland was the first WFN President who worked for closer contact between the WFN and the International Brain Research Organization (IBRO).

Masland and *World Neurology*

Until Masland's presidency, the only available WFN newsletter was the *Journal of the Neurological Sciences*. Masland realized the importance of a separate newsletter with information about the development of the WFN, news from the Research Groups, and communication about activities in the neurosciences worldwide.

The first newsletter of the World Federation of Neurology appeared in 1983 as *Highlights of the Meeting of the Council of Delegates and Research Committee WFN Hamburg*. It contained information not only about the coming World Congress, but also about the WFN Research Groups and the development of the organization. It then appeared in June 1984 (second announcement), November 1984 (third announcement), and as the pre-congress issue on 15 July 1985. The Congress Management and the German Organizing Committee underwrote the cost of the four issues, which were circulated to over 18,000 neurologists.

This might have been the last issue of *World Neurology*, but Masland and the Secretary-Treasurer General, James Toole, managed to keep *World Neurology* going, first distributed by Winston-Salem and published by Raven Press. Number 1, volume 1, was dated April 1988. The 1989 volume (number 3, volume 4) was the last to be published by Winston-Salem. From 1990, Frank Clifford Rose, who had been elected the new Secretary-Treasurer General in New Delhi, took over as the new Editor-in-Chief of *World Neurology* (62).

Several pharmaceutical companies, Eisai, Hoechst Marion Roussel, Schering Healthcare, Lilly, and Smith Kline Beecham, gave substantial grants to help with the costs of publishing *World Neurology* in its new format, first with Eldred Smith-Gordon and subsequently with Cambridge Medical Publications. Frank Clifford Rose was the Editor-in-Chief of *World Neurology* for nine successful years. On 31 December 1998, Richard Godwin-Austen succeeded him as Secretary-Treasurer General, and Professor Jagjit Chopra, India, became the new Editor-in-Chief. Surplus finds from the successful world congress in New Delhi were important during the early 2000s.

When the WFN found it difficult to support *World Neurology*, Lord Walton asked the delegates to look for external sponsorships. In response, Dr Eijiro Satoyoshi arranged for the Eisai Pharmaceutical Company in Japan to support publication for several years. Much later, during Kimura's tenure as WFN President, the WFN again faced a shortage of funds to cover the cost of the journal, in view of expanding allocation of available resources for various educational activities globally. Dr Satoyoshi, after retirement from Toho University, became the head of the Japan Foundation for Neuroscience and Mental Health, which served as a vehicle to support fundraising for various neurological meetings. Having organized a number of national and international conferences with considerable fiscal success, Kimura had deposited the surplus for future academic use in accordance with Japanese governmental regulations. Dr Satoyoshi and Kimura hoped to donate part of this sum to the WFN cause. After a series of negotiations, they were able to divert US$50,000 per year for five years from 2003 through 2007. Thanks to this initiative, using advertisement revenue, the WFN could maintain the publication of *World Neurology* until the journal became self-supporting.

John Walton: the WFN comes of age

John Walton (Fig. 2.9) was elected President of the World Federation of Neurology at the World Congress of Neurology in New Delhi in 1989. The new President knew the organization from the inside better than anyone else. He had saved the WFN with his compromise during the WANC crisis in 1966. He had started the Research Group on Neuromuscular Disorders and had been Chairman of the Research Committee. He had been Editor-in-Chief of the *Journal of the Clinical Neurosciences*. He was First Vice President of the WFN during Masland's presidency. He also chaired the Committee on Constitution & Bye-laws.

Walton had Frank Clifford Rose (London, UK) as Secretary-Treasurer General. Klaus Poeck (Achen, Germany) was elected First Vice President and Chairman of the Research Committee. Other Vice Presidents were Art Asbury (USA), Ben Hamida (Tunisia), James W. Lance (Australia), Alberto Portera Sanchez (Spain), and Noshir Wadia (India).

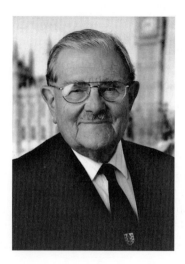

Fig. 2.9 John Walton, the fifth WFN President. The WFN comes of age.

Courtesy of Lord Walton.

THE SHAPING OF THE ORGANIZATION | **59**

John Nicholas Walton was born in Rowlands Gill near Durham, UK, in 1922, the son of a teacher. He trained at King's College in the University of Durham, now the University of Newcastle-upon-Tyne, where he graduated in 1945 with First Class Honours and Distinctions in Medicine, Surgery, and Midwifery. During National Service he served in the Western Approaches and the Middle East, later joining the Territorial Army. He became a medical registrar at the Royal Victoria Infirmary in Newcastle, and demonstrated his potential for research and writing through his MD thesis on subarachnoid haemorrhage, on which Professor Nattrass and Sir Charles Symonds examined him, and which he later turned into an outstanding book in 1956. He was persuaded by Nattrass and Henry Miller to forgo an initial interest in paediatrics. In 1951 he became a research assistant and worked first at the National Hospital, Queen Square, to study neurophysiology, especially electromyography. In 1953, he went to the USA to do research in muscle disorders with Professor Ray Adams at the Massachusetts General Hospital in Boston, before writing his second book, a comprehensive text on polymyositis, the start of his lifelong interest in muscle disease. His phenotypic classification of muscle disease laid the foundation for subsequent studies in molecular genetics. He became the head of the neurology department and initiated the establishment of the Muscular Dystrophy Laboratories in Newcastle, which became internationally known for its research into neuromuscular diseases.

In 1961 he wrote the book that became a standard text for medical students, *Essentials of Neurology*. In 1964 he edited the first edition of *Disorders of Voluntary Muscle* and in 1969, shortly after his appointment as Professor, he was invited to follow Lord Brain as author of *Diseases of the Nervous System*.

In 1968, he was promoted to a personal chair in neurology, and in 1971 appointed the Dean of Medicine at Newcastle-upon-Tyne, a post which he held for a decade and during which he was knighted. John Walton was President of the British Medical Association from 1980 to 1982, President of the General Medical Council 1982 to 1989 and President of the Royal Society of Medicine from 1984 to 1986. From 1983 to 1989 he was Warden of Green College, Oxford—the sister College of St Edmund's College, Cambridge, and moved from Newcastle to Oxford in 1983.

In Europe, a Pan-European Society of Neurology had already been formed, and at John Walton's proposal it became the European Federation of Neurological Societies under the auspices of the WFN at the Pan-European Congress in Vienna in 1991. John Walton is an Honorary Member of the EFNS.

He was knighted in 1979 and was created a life peer in 1989 as Baron Walton of Detchant, of Detchant in the County of Northumberland, and sits as a crossbencher. He has contributed to debates in the House of Lords, particularly the Human Fertilisation and Embryology Bill. His work in the House of Lords continues. His opinion is respected, whenever medical, scientific, or educational matters are discussed and he has served as a member and chairman of several important committees and reports (36).

The World 1989–1997: German reunification, Nelson Mandela, and the Bosnian War—the decade of the brain

German reunification in 1990 was the process in which the German Democratic Republic and a reunited Berlin joined the Federal Republic of Germany. Nelson Mandela was released in 1990, signalling the beginning of a transition to democracy in South Africa. In 1994, he was elected President of South Africa.

Iraq invaded Kuwait in 1990. The break up of Yugoslavia (Bosnian War) began in 1992. Bill Clinton was elected President of the USA in 1992. In 1990, the US Congress signed a bill on 'The Decade of the Brain'.

In 1976, Baruch S. Blumberg and D. Carleton Gajdusek shared the Nobel Prize for their work on kuru and Creutzfeldt–Jacob disease. Twenty years after Gajdusek, neurosciences had exploded, and the Nobel Prize in Physiology or Medicine 1997 was awarded to Stanley B. Prusiner for his discovery of prions—a new biological principle of infection.

Walton's presidency

More than 30 years had passed since the WFN had been founded in Brussels in 1957. The WFN now had to face the challenges of a new time. The organization had grown considerably, with increasing demands upon the Federation. It needed professionalism, but that would also require structural changes to the organization.

Walton's presidency became the most constructive modernization phase in the history of the WFN. It lasted during Walton and Toole's Presidencies, and some of the last elements of the reorganization were first brought in place during Kimura's presidency. The reason why the process took such time is that thorough discussion was essential in order to mobilize the members in the modernization process. Walton took care that the changes were constitutional and carried through by the WFN National Delegates and the WFN Committees, and that all WFN members were informed about the process.

Walton and Rose decided to invite management consultants from the UK Charities Aid Foundation (CAF) to advise on changes for modernizing the governance of the organization (63). Their recommendations have had far-reaching consequences for the Federation, and are therefore presented in detail.

The modernization of the WFN governance

In their evaluation, the CAF consultants concluded that the committee structure largely prescribed the Federation's committee structure and officers. While amendments have been made over the years, they advised a general revision in due course.

The CAF consultants pointed out that only the Research Committee had written responsibilities and might well entrust executive matters to the Management Committee. These were needed for all the other committees. The large number dealing with internal matters called for review to rationalize the conduct of business. The responsibilities of the Publications and the Continuing Education Committees needed reinforcement. Working parties were encouraged to further the Federation's cause, under the general direction of the First Vice President. How to increase income to create means for meetings at a distance needed to be explored.

Defining the responsibilities of the First Vice President would ease pressure on the President. It was also recommended to separate the offices of the Secretary-General and Treasurer, because this would spread work and build in safeguards. So far, this separation has not been performed, mainly because the Management Committee saw that it might complicate and delay work, and has therefore decided to have close collaboration between the Secretary-Treasurer General and the Chair of the WFN Finance Committee.

One of the most central steps of reorganization was to establish corporate status for the WFN. Registration as a UK company limited by guarantee was advisable to reassure the Charity Commissioners for England and Wales if at any times questions should be raised about the majority of Trustees being resident in other countries in the future. The impending appointment of officers based in different countries and continents made the creation of a new Secretariat pressing. The CAF consultants pointed out that the responsibilities of the Management Committee as 'Trustees' in United Kingdom law must be understood and respected, and responsibilities clearly assigned to it. A collegiate model was favoured, housed in a suitable parent body, which would be able to provide back-up services.

The list of recommendations can be summarized as follows:

1 The Publications Committee to be strengthened.

2 The establishment of an integrated secretariat.

3 Costs of establishing and maintaining the new Secretariat to be a primary claim upon income from financial reserves.

4 Financial planning systems, including itemized annual budgets, to be introduced and expenditure monitored to the Treasurer and reported to the Finance Committee.

5 The Management Committee to explore the feasibility of housing the new Secretariat in a suitable collegiate environment, with support services.

6 The new Editor of the newsletter to commission market research to inform future editorial policy and content.

7 The Committee structure to be reviewed.

8 Responsibilities of committees be agreed in writing.

9 The Research Committee to invite the Management Committee to handle extensive matters on its behalf.

10 The Continuing Education Committee to be strengthened.

11 Working parties to be established to promote and develop aspects of the Federation's work.

12 The Federation to separate the offices of Secretary-General and Treasurer.

13 The Constitution to be reviewed once the above recommendations had been considered.

The internal discussion in the WFN

The report from the CAF consultants was presented to the Management Committee. The accounts of the WFN were now healthy (64). With minor changes, the WFN delegates decided to apply to change the status of the organization to that of a charity (65).

First, the report was discussed with the Management Committee during the American Academy of Neurology (AAN) meeting in San Francisco in March 1996. It was then published in *World Neurology* in September 1996, presented to the national WFN delegates, and discussed at the Council of Delegates in Buenos Aires in 1997 (63).

The WFN had submitted a preliminary application for charity status in 1993, but it was clear that the organization first needed to modernize its governance. In 1995, the WFN was accepted as a charity organization under UK law, and the decision was given retrospectively to 1991. One consequence of the decision was that if the WFN were registered as a charity, it would also be able to accept tax-deductible donations (64). As a consequence, tax paid was reimbursed for the period 1991–1995.

Putting advice into action

One recommendation was that the responsibilities of the Committees be defined. The Chairs of the Publications and of the Finance Committees were contacted and their responsibilities defined (see 'The Modernization of the WFN governance', p. 61). Jun Kimura (Chairman of the Constitution & Bye-laws Committee), Robert Daroff (Chairman of the Publications

Committee), Ted Munsat (Chairman of the Research and Continuing Education Committee), and Richard Godwin-Austen (Secretary-Treasurer General) began initiating and developing a full range of activities and projects for their committees (67–69).

A permanent WFN Secretariat

The consultants pointed out that the location of the Secretariat was a matter for the Federation, but found advantages in remaining in the UK. A permanent secretariat was established at 12 Chandos Street, London, UK, in the building owned by the Medical Society of London, and Mr Keith Newton began his employment as Administrator of the Federation (66, 67). The premises were at first a little cramped, but in 2008 the Secretariat moved to modern premises at Richmond, Surrey.

There were counter-arguments against a permanent WFN Secretariat, and there were arguments for moving the WFN headquarters every four years. It was, however, decided during the WFN Congress in Buenos Aires in 1997 to stabilize the administrative functions using a permanent Secretariat to co-ordinate and implement this work. It was fitting that the first World Congress of the new millennium should be held in London in line with the recommendations of the CAF as approved by the Council of Delegates (68, 69).

The Administrator is a key person in the Federation. Keith Newton has a broad background in the administration of national medical organizations and under his able leadership, the historic continuity of the WFN is preserved and activities are formally evaluated in relation to the Articles of Association. He maintains the WFN database, provides the auditor with necessary accounts, and maintains financial records. He assists the Secretary-General in executing decisions by the Council of Delegates, arranges meetings of the Council and Committees, and deals with correspondence within, and/or on behalf of, the WFN.

The Decade of the Brain

The US Congress, in concert with President George Bush, declared the 1990s the 'Decade of the Brain'. In response to a request by the US Congress, the Advisory Council of the National Institute of Neurological Disorders and Stroke produced an implementation plan, focusing on 14 major disease categories in which neurological research gives promise of rapid progress for the coming decade. The plan called for increased allocations to basic and clinical neurosciences of $190 million in the first year, rising to $385 million per year in the latter part of the decade. Dr G. M. McKhann chaired the implementation panel (70).

The House of Representatives Joint Resolution 174 declaring the 1990s as the 'Decade of the Brain' also made it urgent to obtain a commitment from neurologists all over the world. At the meeting of the Council of Delegates in New Delhi in 1989, the WFN strongly endorsed the action of the US Congress and encouraged its other members to urge their national governing bodies to pass similar resolutions. Several national neurological societies, in Europe and elsewhere, celebrated the 'Decade of the Brain' throughout the 1990s to substantiate the progress in clinical and basic neurosciences.

Clinical neurophysiology

For a long time, there had been resistance to the idea of deliberately expanding the scope of clinical neurophysiology, but in 1990 the International Federation of Societies of EEG and Clinical Neurophysiology was renamed the International Federation of Clinical Neurophysiology. The new name acknowledged the equal importance of EEG and EMG (67). Although the renaming had nothing directly to do with the WFN, the consequences were clear for most practising neurologists, reflecting the equal importance of EEG and EMG, and the unity of clinical neurophysiology as one discipline.

The WFN and the WHO

It was during Walton's presidency that the head of the Division of Mental Health of the WHO, Norman Sartorius, invited the leaders of the non-governmental organizations (NGOs) in neurosciences to an annual meeting towards the end of the year. This became an important door opener for future contacts and subsequent collaboration between the WFN and the WHO.

James Toole: a new WFN

The Council of Delegates in Buenos Aires elected James Toole WFN President in 1997 (Fig. 2.10). He was the first WFN President who to be elected for one period (four years) only. Like Walton, Toole also knows the WFN from the inside. He was the WFN Secretary-Treasurer General in Masland's administration, 1981–1989. Together with Masland, he enabled the new WFN Newsletter, *World Neurology*, to survive, and it has become an important communication medium for the Federation. In 1989, Toole became the Editor-in-Chief of the *Journal of Neurological Sciences*.

In Toole's administration, Jun Kimura (Kyoto, Japan) was elected First Vice President, and Richard Godwin-Austen (London, UK) Secretary-Treasurer General.

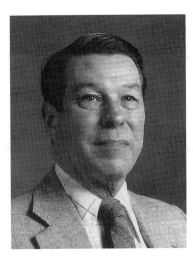

Fig. 2.10 James Toole, the sixth WFN President. A new WFN.

Courtesy of James Toole.

James F. Toole was born in Atlanta, Georgia, in 1925. He received his BA degree from Princeton University in 1947, his MD degree from Cornell University Medical College in 1949, and his LLB from LaSalle Extension University in 1963. From 1948 to 1958, he did his postgraduate training in Havana (Cuba), Philadelphia, Pennsylvania, and at the Institute of Neurology, Queen Square, London, as a Fulbright scholar. The American Board of Internal Medicine, American Board of Psychiatry and Neurology, American Society of Neuroimaging–Neurosonology, and the American Board of Neurorehabilitation, certify him. Toole was Chairman of the Department of Neurology at the Bowman Gray School of Medicine, Winston Salem, North Carolina, from 1962 to 1983 and was the Walter C. Teagle Professor of Neurology for 45 years and Director of the Cerebrovascular Research Center. Toole has special insight and competence in cerebrovascular disorders. He started work on his book *Cerebrovascular Disorders* in 1964, and it is now (2012) in its 6th edition (72).

The world 1997–2001: Hong Kong; September 11

In 1997, Hong Kong, the former British colony, became an integral part of the People's Republic of China. The attacks on the Pentagon in Washington and the World Trade Center in New York took place on 11 September 2001.

The Nobel Prize in Physiology or Medicine for 2000 was awarded jointly to three neuroscientists, Arvid Carlsson, Paul Greengard, and Eric R. Kandel, for their discoveries concerning signal transduction in the nervous system.

66 | THE HISTORY OF THE WORLD FEDERATION OF NEUROLOGY

James Toole's presidency

Many of the decisions taken by the Council of Delegates during the 1990s were implemented during Toole's administration. He organized the Ad-hoc Strategic Planning group meeting at Sopwell House Hotel, St Albans, UK, in 1999. This was important, because the WFN national delegates could meet here to evaluate the structure of the Federation after 10 years of constructive reorganization (73).

Ad-hoc Strategic Planning Group Meeting at Sopwell House

From 1957, there had been numerous discussions on the WFN mission. It had also been discussed at St Albans, and it was now changed to read: It shall be the purpose of the World Federation of Neurology to improve human health worldwide by promoting prevention and the care of persons with disorders of the entire nervous system by:

- Fostering the best standards of neurological practice.
- Educating, in collaboration with neuroscience and other international public and private organizations.
- Facilitating research through its Research Groups and other means.

The proposed mission statement emphasized that the primary purpose of the WFN is to improve the health of people, and it focused on standards, education, and research.

Reorganization/construction of the WFN

The organization of the WFN has often been reconsidered, and the Ad-hoc Strategic Planning Group at Sopwell House recommended that:

1 The WFN be governed by a Board of Directors to include a President, Vice President, Secretary-Treasurer General, Research Committee Chair, and three Directors-at-large, all elected by the Council of Delegates from nominations proposed either by the Nominating Committee or by five members of the Council of Delegates, with sufficient advance notice, and the five regional Presidents.

2 The terms of office generally be four years.

3 A Management Committee (by 2000 renamed Trustees) of officers to exist for immediate decision-making.

4 Countries to continue to be members (with some exceptions as approved by the Directors) with Delegates elected/chosen by the National Neurological Societies.

5 Standing Committees of the Directors (e.g. Finance, Bye-laws, Research, etc.) and Operating Committees (e.g. Education, Public Relations, Publications, etc.) to be approved by the President with the approval of the Directors.

The group then discussed strategic goals and directions. There was a full agreement that the Research Groups should continue to play a central role in the WFN activities. The individual Research Committee Statutes were abolished when the Research Committee became a Standing Committee of the WFN.

It was also agreed that the aim of WFN's educational activities should focus priority on neurological health problems that have been identified. There has been full agreement that effective medical education is a primary concern and need. Under the leadership of Theodore Munsat, Chair of the new WFN Research and Continuing Education Committee, the WFN initiated a series of 1-year pilot studies using the American Academy of Neurology programme *Continuum*. The idea is that the participating national neurological societies select 20 neurologists, all from the same region, who then take four specially designed courses. The long-term aim of the pilot programmes is to establish regular discussion groups focused on maintaining up-to-date practice skills in an age of rapidly increasing information (74).

WFN Council of Delegates

Two important WFN meetings took place in 2000 and 2001 (75,76). The WFN Council of Delegates met in May 2000. In September, the Trustees began the final phase in establishing the corporate status. The Council of Delegates completed this during the 2001 World Congress in London. The Memorandum and Articles of Association were then formally adopted.

The meeting of the Council of Delegates in London on 17 June 2001 was a historic event for the WFN. It marked the formal dissolution of the 'old' organization and the transfer of its finances and other assets to the incorporated WFN that had co-existed alongside its namesake for the last three years of Toole's presidency.

Formal transition to corporate status

James Toole's administration worked with tremendous speed and efficiency. The first part of the process was to identify all revisions approved by the Council of Delegates after 1990 to make the document consistent with the current rules under which WFN operated. The key person in this process was the new First Vice President, Jun Kimura, who was also the Chair of the Constitution & Bye-laws Committee. Dianne C. Vernon was executive assistant. The final version was distributed among the Delegates of the WFN on 6 January 1999 as the current policy in practice.

With the formal adoption of the Memorandum and Articles of Association, the final phase in establishing corporate status was initiated. It included dissolving the old WFN, and transferring all of its membership and assets to WFN Inc. under the endorsement of the UK Charity Commission. This carefully planned process was completed during the London Congress, thus marking a new era for the WFN. The transition came to fruition during Toole's presidency, five years after the project was initiated by the previous administration.

The responsibilities of the Publications Committee were clarified and strengthened during Toole's presidency. A number of key procedures and policy areas were formulated in accordance with the Federation's Memorandum and Articles of Association, now that its incorporation as a company under UK law had been formally achieved (see Appendix 1).

The relationship with the WHO was also discussed at the Planning Meeting and it was agreed that the WFN should increase its contact and influence with the WHO, but one unresolved issue remained, should there be a WHO position representing neurology funded by the WFN? That WHO position came in 2008.

Jun Kimura: the first WFN President from outside the western world

Jun Kimura (Fig. 2.11) was the First Vice President in James Toole's administration. He also chaired the Constitution & Bye-laws Committee during the critical transition period from the 'old' organization to the incorporated WFN.

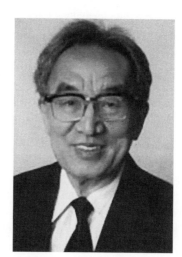

Fig. 2.11 Jun Kimura, the seventh WFN President. The first WFN President from outside the western world.

Courtesy of Jun Kimura.

Johan Aarli (Bergen, Norway) was elected First Vice President in Kimura's administration. The post of Secretary-Treasurer General was not contested on this occasion, and Richard Godwin-Austen remained in this position. Julien Bogousslavsky (Lausanne, Switzerland), William Carroll (Perth, Australia), and Roberto Sica (Buenos Aires, Argentina) were elected Trustees. Jin Soo Kim (South Korea) was elected Regional Vice President for the Asian-Oceanian region, Leontino Battistin (Italy) for the European, Najoua Miladi (Tunisia) for the Pan-African, Pedro Chana (Chile) and Carlos Chouza (Uruguay) for the Pan-American, and S. Al Deeb (Saudi Arabia) for the Pan-Arab region. From 2005 on, the Regional Presidents were elected as Regional Directors by the Regional Associations and appointed by the Council of Delegates.

According to the new constitution, the three Elected Trustees took up their duties with immediate effect, while all others began their terms of office on 1 January 2002. Kimura appointed Theodore Munsat as Co-opted Trustee and Chair of the WFN Education Committee. Roger Rosenberg was the Chair of the Research Committee. In 2002, Marianne de Visser was elected Trustee for a three-year term. She was re-elected in 2005, and served successfully as the Chair of the WFN Membership Committee.

Jun Kimura received a Bachelor of Technology degree in 1957 and MD in 1961 from Kyoto University in Japan. He moved to the USA as a Fulbright scholar in 1962 for residency training in neurology and fellowship in electrophysiology at the University of Iowa. He taught at the University of Manitoba in Canada, the University of Iowa in the USA, Kyoto University in Japan, and Tiantan Hospital in China. He served as President of the International Federation of Clinical Neurophysiology (IFCN) and the World Federation of Neurology (WFN), and as Editor-in-Chief of *Muscle & Nerve*.

Working as a clinical neurologist, Dr Kimura has a special interest in neuromuscular disorders in general and clinical electrophysiology in particular. His book *Electrodiagnosis in Diseases of Nerve and Muscle* has appeared in four editions. He has received an honorary membership from 25 national societies of neurology, neurophysiology, and rehabilitation medicine.

The World 2001–2005: Invasion of Iraq and war in Afghanistan

Two wars dominated world news during this period. The war in Afghanistan was launched in response to the 9/11 attacks, and the Iraq War began in 2003 with the invasion of Iraq.

The Nobel Prize in medicine and physiology for 2003 was awarded to Paul C. Lauterbur (USA) and Sir Peter Mansfield (UK) for their discoveries concerning magnetic resonance imaging.

Kimura's presidency

During Toole's administration, the final phase in establishing the corporate status of the WFN had been accomplished. In addition to being the First Vice President during Toole's presidency, Kimura chaired the Constitution & Bye-laws Committee, whose main function was to update the WFN structure so it could become compatible with current policies and practices. Thanks to Kimura's skills and insight in the organization, the transition was so smooth that many national delegates did not notice any major difference in the WFN function, although many of the basic elements of the Federation now had obtained a new structure.

The Constitution & Bye-laws Committee decided to tackle this revision in two tiers. The first stage consisted of adding all the changes already approved by the Council of Delegates (COD) after the New Delhi Congress, when the previous version of the Constitution & Bye-laws was produced. The second stage was to make further radical modifications to ensure that all practices were fully compatible with the Articles of Association now that the WFN was to be incorporated under UK law as a company limited by guarantee. Gathering the information for the first step proved to be easier said than done, primarily because we had to locate the specific wording of the modifications that were scattered in different documents over the span of 10 years. Recent personnel changes within the organization and the relocation of the Secretariat also made it difficult to pinpoint the exact source of information. With help from the members of the Executive Committee and Keith Newton at the London office, however, all papers pertinent for revision were collected.

Production of the updated documents completed the first stage of the review of the current status of the WFN (77). The first draft was circulated among the members of the Committee on 3 August 1998, followed by the second and third drafts on 15 September and 7 December after appropriate amendments based on various suggestions received. With the approval of the Executive Committee, the final version was forwarded to the Secretariat for printing. The document was then distributed among the Delegates of the WFN on 6 January 1999 as the current policy in practice. As stated earlier, incorporated in this draft were all the revisions approved by the Council of Delegates after 1990, when the last version was printed. Thus, this first stage of 'revision' was simply a 'catch-up' process to make the document consistent with the current rules under which we operated. No changes were incorporated except for the clauses necessary for the provisions with the Charity Commission. The references included 1991, 1993, 1995, and 1997 COD, and Memorandum of Association and Articles of Association under the Companies Act 1985 and 1989 of the United Kingdom.

The formal adoption of the Memorandum and Articles of Association initiated the final phase in establishing corporate status, dissolving the old WFN, and transferring all of its membership and assets to WFN Inc. under the endorsement of the UK Charity Commission. This carefully planned process was completed during the London Congress in 2001, thus marking a new era for our Federation. The transition came to fruition under the leadership of President James Toole, five years after the project was initiated by the previous administration.

Jun Kimura was elected as the next President of Federation at this important juncture. Kimura's presidency was the first period in the history of the Federation when a new and modernized structure was applied. When his presidency was finished, WFN had achieved the missions and objectives of the newly incorporated Federation. The new WFN could now meet the challenges of the modern world. The old WFN was dissolved. All of its membership and assets were transferred to WFN Inc. under the endorsement of the UK Charity Commission (78).

Kimura decided to keep all the existing Committees with the exception of Neuroethics, which was reconstituted as the 'Neuroethics Research Group' because of its inherent nature. The Public Relations Committee was renamed the Public Relations and WHO Liaison Committee, and the Continuing Education Committee was named the Education Committee. Kimura adopted a policy of rotating most committee chairmen off their positions and nominating new people to take their place, with the exception of the Education (Munsat) and the Public Relations and WHO Liaison (Aarli) Committees.

The first test of the new structure was the annual Council of Delegates 2002.

Vancouver 2002: Testing the new Articles of Association

Previously, the WFN Council of Delegates had met every two years, once during the quadrennial World Congress of Neurology and the other during the preplanning meeting for the next World Congress. During the restructuring process associated with the WFN being incorporated it was decided that the meetings of the Council of Delegates should be held annually. The first annual general meeting had already taken place in London in 1999.

Some colleagues had expressed concern about the strict rules, particularly the need for annual meetings. Kimura also wondered whether the UK's regulations would allow the flexibility necessary for an international organization. In these days of modern communication, some saw no point in asking people to travel long distances, at great expense, for a few hours at a meeting. Kimura's administration, however, opted to give a little more time to test the new Articles of Association, which were only one year old. Besides, the new rules had a number of features he would like to exploit, such as tax exemption, fund raising, and protection of the WFN from liability. Also, most clauses, intentionally written 'loosely' without specifics, allowed the administration to conduct day-to-day operation according to the policy manual that could be readily modified based on changing needs.

The first Annual General Meeting after the new constitution went into effect, on 7 July 2002, at the time of the Xth International Congress on Neuromuscular Diseases in Vancouver. There had been some concerns about adequate delegate attendance because the WFN had no previous experience of calling the Council of Delegates only one year after the World Congress of Neurology. Although some 34 member societies initially indicated their participation, only 24 representatives eventually attended, with four additional countries offering a proxy assigned to a delegate of their choice. To compound the problem, most countries were represented by one of the attendees of the Neuromuscular Congress rather than the registered national delegate, and the participants revealed their interest and insight in the new constitution. The Council of Delegates was well organized, and one advantage was that none of the issues discussed were delayed and that the agenda was updated. Marianne de Visser was elected as a new Trustee (78).

With the completion of Kimura's presidency at the end of 2005, there was agreement that the Federation had obtained a structure that was adapted to meet the challenges of the future.

The new Federation centred on improving health worldwide by promoting education and research in neurology as well as the prevention and treatment of disorders of the nervous system. Some of the main goals included (1) establishing the Secretariat in London to facilitate interaction with its members under the care of our administrator, Mr Keith Newton, with the assistance of Ms Susan Bilger; (2) facilitating international programmes under the direction of Ted Munsat as the Chair of the Education Committee and Roger Rosenberg as Chair of the Research Committee; (3) initiating comprehensive prospective budgetary controls under the scrutiny of Dr Richard Godwin-Austen as Secretary-Treasurer and Dr Robert Daroff as the Chair of the Finance Committee; and (4) formulating goal-oriented long-term plans under the direction of the Steering Committee Chaired by Dr Vladimir Hachinski. Many of these important projects stemmed from the Strategic Planning Meeting held in St Albans in 2000, making steady progress in achieving some of the missions agreed upon during those intense discussions.

Specifically, the WFN tried to encourage and assist the education of young neurologists in developing countries. This would achieve great worldwide recognition of our discipline, and make the prevention and treatment of neurological conditions the number one priority of governmental medical policies.

WFN administration and association management companies

In 2002, Keith Newton brought up an option for the WFN's possible future administrative arrangements, which would involve outsourcing to a professional management company. The International Federation of Clinical Neurophysiology had decided to function in this way, using Concorde Services as their secretariat.

In February 2003, the WFN Structure and Function Committee concluded that using a professional management company would increase flexibility and efficiency, and that fund-raising should be a major part of the project. After careful identification of a dedicated association management company, the risks for the WFN appeared minimal, and obviously smaller than the present risks of dysfunction with the present secretariat/management system. The following companies: Congrex (Concord Services), Ernst and Young, Kenes, and MCI, were discarded by the WFN after perusal of their proposal or visits to their headquarters. Further to the recommendation of the Committee, the WFN then selected two companies, GIC Management (GIC), and Association Global Services (AGS), both based in Brussels.

Drs Kimura, Godwin-Austen, Bogousslavsky, and Aarli visited the two candidate companies in August 2004. The report was presented to the Trustees, and the preliminary information was presented to the WFN Council of Delegates in Paris on 5 September 2004. The delegates approved the Trustees' recommendations, but only pending satisfactory contractual arrangements (79). It soon became clear that the costs with GIC, or with AGS, would be higher than the present London office costs. On this basis, the Trustees decided that involving professional association management companies for administration of the WFN did not offer administrative advantages, and might disturb the present institutional memory, which is essential for the function of the WFN. All the Trustees were very satisfied with the present set-up in the London office, and with the rapid responses they received from the staff there.

The main conclusion was therefore that professional management with GIC (or AGS) would not be pursued for the time being; that the London Office would remain open, and that Miss Bilger would be replaced in due course when her eventual retirement was effected (80).

Johan A. Aarli—the WFN becomes a global organization

Johan Arild Aarli (Fig. 2.12) was elected President of the WFN at the World Congress of Neurology in Sydney 2005. Vladimir Hachinski was elected First

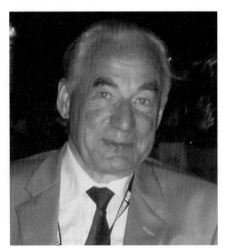

Fig. 2.12 Johan A. Aarli, the eighth WFN President. The WFN becomes a global organization.

Courtesy of Johan A. Aarli.

Vice President. Richard Godwin-Austen remained the Secretary-Treasurer General for one more year, according to the constitution. Julien Bogousslavsky (Lausanne, Switzerland) was re-elected Trustee, and was scheduled to take over as Secretary-Treasurer General from 2007. Owing to financial irregularities at his University in Lausanne, his position became open (81). The Trustees conducted a recount of the votes cast at the election in Sydney and Raad Shakir (London, UK), the second candidate after Julien was elected Secretary-Treasurer General by the Council of Delegates in Glasgow 2006, took over with effect from 1 January 2007 (82).

Johan Arild Aarli was born in Kvinesdal, Norway, in 1936. He graduated in medicine from the University of Bergen in 1961. His career in neurology began in the 1960s, a period marked by dramatic changes in treatment procedures. He did research on experimental myasthenia gravis with Professor Edith Heilbronn at the National Research Institute of Sweden in Stockholm and at the University of Chicago in 1989. He showed that titin is the striatal muscle antigen to which most patients with thymoma and myasthenia gravis have antibodies.

In 1977, he became professor of neurology and head of the department of neurology at the University of Bergen (Norway) Hospital, where he remained until retiring in 2006. He established a spinal unit, a regional epilepsy centre, an amyotrophic lateral sclerosis clinic, a stroke unit, a national multiple sclerosis centre and registry, a myasthenia gravis competence centre, and a neuroimmunology research centre. In 1996 he was knighted by King Harald V and became Knight, First Class, of Saint Olav's Order. He was Vice Dean of the faculty of medicine at the University of Bergen from 1982 to 1984, dean from 1985 to

THE SHAPING OF THE ORGANIZATION | **75**

1987. He is an honorary member of the American Neurological Association, honorary corresponding member of the American Academy of Neurology, and honorary foreign member of the Association of British Neurologists and of the French Society of Neurology.

He was the Chair of the Teaching Committee of the European Federation of Neurological Societies (EFNS) 1997–2002 and EFNS Secretary-General 2003–2005. He became the Norwegian delegate to the WFN in 1991, and chaired the WFN Public Relations Committee from 1995. Under the administrations of WFN Presidents James Toole and Jun Kimura he was the Liaison Officer to the WHO.

The world 2005–2009

Pope John Paul II died in April 2005 and was succeeded by Benedict XVI. Mahmoud Ahmadinejad won the presidential election in Iran. An earthquake in Pakistan killed 80,000 people.

Two international wars, in Iraq and in Afghanistan, were going on in this period, and in 2005, four bombs exploded in London, linked to al Qaeda. The power-sharing agreement for Northern Ireland was signed in 2007.

Aarli's presidency

Aarli had two main initiatives as President of the WFN. First, he articulated the need to study and develop new and creative methods to implement improved delivery and increased rural distribution of neurological health, his 'The Africa Initiative'. He started this initiative in 2005 and it was his primary mission statement when being considered for President (83). Second, he was determined to bring into the WFN the 1.2 billion people within the People's Republic of China. By virtue of his persistent diplomatic manner and style, he was able to implement successfully both initiatives.

Under the leadership of Benedetto Saraceno and his successor Shekhar Saxena at the Department of Mental Health in the WHO, the collaboration between the WFN and WHO improved considerably. Aarli initiated the close relationship and collaboration between the WFN and the Department of Mental Health at the WHO, and Tarun Dua, MD, a specialist in paediatric neurology, became the first neurologist associated with the WHO (84).

When Johan Aarli was elected First Vice President in 2001, he initiated a discussion on the relationship between the WFN central administration and the Regional Vice Presidents. By 2003, the Trustees had arrived at a new definition of the Regional Directors, which was approved by the WFN Council of Delegates. This is further described in Chapter 6 about the Regional Neurological Associations.

A closer contact with the WHO: the neurology atlas— a torch for Africa

Aarli's administration focused upon Africa simply because Africa confronted the world's most dramatic public health crisis. There was general agreement on a policy to work out a roadmap for developing neurology in Africa at the WFN Strategy meeting in San Diego in 2006.

The WFN Africa programme was launched at a meeting in London in December 2006 where Dr Jose Bertolote, the Vice Director for the Department of Mental Health, represented the WHO and discussed future collaboration between the WHO and the WFN. The work and recommendations were then developed together with African colleagues, especially Redda T. Haimanot (Ethiopia), Pierre Bill (Durban, South Africa), Amadou Gallo Diop (Dakar, Senegal), and Michel Dumas (Limoges, France).

At the London meeting, a Task and Advisory Force for Neurology in Africa (TAFNA), chaired by Amadou Gallo Diop and Johan Aarli, was established. Rajesh Kalaria represents a link with IBRO and SONA (Society of Neuroscientists of Africa). Gallo Diop is setting up the WFN Africa Committee with African neurologists working and residing in the continent.

Training of neurologists for Africa

The first meeting of the newly established WFN Africa Committee was held in Stellenbosch, South Africa, in 2008 with the following African colleagues: Chafiq Hicham (Morocco), Melaku Zenebe (Ethiopia), Pierre Bill (South Africa), Elly Katabira (Uganda), Mohamed Arezki (Algeria), Amadou Gallo Diop (Senegal), Beugre Kouassi (Ivory Coast), Alfred Njamnshi (Cameroon), Girish Modi (South Africa), and Erastus Amayo (Kenya). Raad Shakir, Keith Newton, and Johan Aarli represented the WFN.

Neurologists from Africa can receive specialty training in South Africa or Senegal. The Pan Arab Union of Neurological Societies (PAUNS) has been helpful in preparing training centres in Morocco and Egypt. An agreement with Cairo University was established in 2010. The initiative was made possible by the efforts of Professor Mohamed S. El-Tamawy, president of the Egyptian Society of Neurology, Psychiatry, and Neurosurgery. They signed a memorandum of understanding for setting up a pilot training programme, which, if successful, could be rolled out elsewhere in Africa. The agreement set the seal on an initiative that began during Aarli's presidency when Dr Ragnar Stien of the University of Oslo, Norway, went to Cairo on a fact-finding mission. The three-year programme is intended for doctors from elsewhere in Africa who will join the Cairo University training programme.

Slow boat to China

In 2007, the Chinese Neurological Society became a member of the WFN (Fig. 2.13). With the most populous state in the world, the People's Republic of China, with over 1.3 billion citizens, on board, the WFN had become a global organization.

China has been a member of the United Nations and of the United Nations Security Council since 1971. The WHO is a UN association and Taiwan is not a WHO member. The WFN is a non-governmental organization, and the Taiwanese Neurological Society has been a member of the WFN since 1965. Unfortunately, at the Kyoto congress in 1981, the delegates from Taiwan were provided with name badges upon which 'Republic of China' appeared. As a reaction, congress participants from mainland China walked out and played no further part in the meeting. In Hamburg in 1985, there were name badges with 'Chinese Republic (Beijing)' and 'ROC (Taiwan)', which seemed to satisfy the delegates.

Two former WFN Presidents, Lord Walton, and Jun Kimura, had had negotiations with the board of the Chinese Neurological Society, discussing WFN membership, but no application for membership had been received. In June 2007, Aarli wrote to the Chairman of the Chinese Neurological Society, Professor Chuan-Zhen Lu of Shanghai, inviting him to apply for Chinese WFN membership:

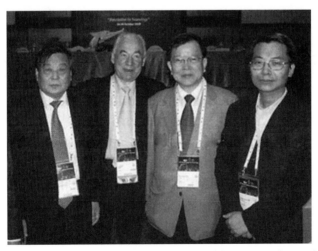

Fig. 2.13 'WE ARE FRIENDS NOW!' From the 19th World Congress of Neurology in Bangkok 2009. From left: Chuan-Zhen Lu from China; WFN President Johan A. Aarli; Ching-Piao Tsai from Taiwan and Raymond Cheung from Hong Kong.

Source: *World Neurol* 24:6. December 2009. Page 7.

I write to you in my capacity of being the President of the World Federation of Neurology (WFN). Unfortunately, China is not a member of this important organization, which I regret very much. Having China as a member would mean much to WFN, to the development of neurology in Asia and to international neurology.

Aarli pointed out that the next World Congress in Neurology would take place in Bangkok, Thailand, in 2009, that Chinese neurology has presented advanced research in world neurology, and that he would like to see Chinese neurologists as speakers in Bangkok.

It is therefore my pleasure and honour to hereby invite the Chinese Neurological Society to become a member nation of the World Federation of Neurology. May I also refer to the WFN Memorandum and Articles of Association for the organization, which is published on the Internet? I am prepared to come to China to discuss the matter of membership and share with you some of our present most important issues, such as the Africa programme, our collaboration with the World Health Organization and the collaboration with psychiatry.

Following positive signals from Chuan-Zhen Lu, Johan Aarli and Raad Shakir as Secretary-Treasurer General of the WFN, wrote the following invitation:

Chinese Neurological Society application for WFN Membership:

The World Federation of Neurology (WFN) welcomes the application of the Chinese Neurological Society to become a member. The WFN is a federation of societies; we, on behalf of the WFN, fully accept that there will be three neurological societies in the China region.

This arrangement is currently acceptable for the World Federation of Neurosurgical Societies, where three societies are represented (the Neurosurgical Society of the People's Republic of China; the Hong Kong Neurosurgical Society; and the Taiwan Neurosurgical Society) and will be acceptable to the WFN.

Whilst we fully understand and are prepared to work with the one China policy, we the WFN, as a WHO accredited organization, will need to follow the same disclaimer produced by the WHO, Regional Office for the western Pacific, July 2004. This states clearly that the designations employed and the presentation of the country and subnational administrative boundary data and other geospatial data do not imply the expression of any opinion whatsoever on the part of the WHO (WFN) concerning the legal status of any country, territory, city or area or of its authorities, or concerning the delimitation of its frontiers or boundaries.

Full WFN membership will allow the Chinese Neurological Society to fully participate in the activities of the WFN, including its Continuing Medical Education Programme; membership of 30 Research Groups; participation in regional and international committees of the WFN; and application to hold Regional Congresses and the World Congress of Neurology in years to come.

We will be happy to co-sign this document with the Chinese Neurological Society.

The board of the Chinese Neurological Society found this a realistic basis for further discussion. Johan Aarli and Raad Shakir flew to Shanghai on 8 August 2007 to discuss with them and sign the document.

The meeting took place 9 August 2007, in a beautiful house in the garden of the Hua Shan Hospital. The host was Mr Liu Zhi, a senior official from the Chinese Medical Association, Beijing. The hospital Director, Mr Hejian Zou, attended the meeting. Professor Lu and the incoming President of the Chinese Neurological Society, Liying Chi, had also come from Beijing for the conference. During the discussion, which took more than four hours, Liu Zhi had several telephone contacts with his department and returned with comments like 'this cannot be accepted'. It was evident that Mr Liu Zhi was well updated and that he knew the history of the WFN very well.

A major issue was that we had grouped the three neurological societies as 'Chinese neurological societies'–China, Hong Kong, and Taiwan—analogous to, for example, 'Scandinavian neurological societies'. After successful agreement, our Chinese hosts invited us for a superb lunch and later for supper after a tour at the Shanghai Museum, where we enjoyed an exhibition of hanging scrolls from the Ming dynasty. It was our pleasure to welcome the Chinese Neurological Society to the WFN.

The Council of Delegates of the WFN convened in Brussels, Belgium, on 26 August 2007, for the Golden Jubilee of the WFN. The Chinese Neurological Society, the neurological societies of The Republic of Congo, Iran, Libya, Nigeria, and Senegal were approved as new members, and the number of members increased to 113.

After the ceremony in Brussels, Aarli assured the Chairman of the Taiwanese Neurological Society, Professor Ching-Kuan Liu, that the society would remain an independent member society of the WFN with its own representation and that the Taiwanese Neurological Society remained in very good standing within the organization.

As a show of unity and a symbol of the understanding reached, the Delegates of the Chinese Neurological Society, the Hong Kong Neurological Society, and the Taiwanese Neurological Society during the subsequent World Congress of Neurology in 2009 were photographed with the President as close friends. When the Chinese Delegate was unable to attend the Council of Delegates in Geneva in 2010, the Delegate from Taiwan, Ching-Piao Tsai, had the proxy from China. The Chinese Neurological Society is now a member of the Asian-Oceanian Association of Neurology, and the World Federation of Neurology has become a global organization (85).

References

1 **Bailey P.** NINDB: origins, founding, and early years (1950–9). In Brady RO, Ed. *The Basic Neurosciences*, vol. 1 of Tower, DB, *The Nervous System*. A Three-Volume Work Commemorating the 25th Anniversary of the National Institute of Neurological and Communicative Disorders and Stroke. New York, Raven Press, 1975, xxi–xxxii.

2 **Rowland LP.** *NINDS at 50.* NIH Publications 01–4161, 2001. Demos Press. New York 2003.

3 **Farreras IG.** 'Establishment of the National Institute of Neurological Diseases and Blindness.' In Farreras IG, Hannaway C, and Harden VA, Eds. *Mind, Brain, Body, and Behavior: Foundations of Neuroscience and Behavioral Research at the National Institutes of Health.* Amsterdam: IOS Press.

4 **Cohen MM,** Presidents of the American Academy of Neurology, *The American Academy of Neurology: The first 50 years, 1949–1998.* American Academy of Neurology.

5 **Poser CM.** The World Federation of Neurology: the formative period 1955–1961. Personal recollections. *J Neur Sci* 1993; **120**: 218–27.

6 **Poser CM.** Personal communications. 2009–2010.

7 **Martin J-J and L.** Hommage à Monsieur Ludo van Bogaert. *Acta Neurol Belg* 1990; **90**: 27–45.

8 **Martin L and J-J.** Ludo van Bogaert (1987–1989). *Acta Neurol Belg* 1996; **96**: 254–63.

9 **Baeck E.** *Ludo van Bogaert (1897–1989) Neurologist, Bibliophile and Patron of the Arts.* 2003; UCB Pharma, Brussels.

10 **Van Bogaert L.** Presidential Report. *J Neur Sci* 1966; **3**: 444–50.

11 **Bailey P.** Report of the meeting of the WFN Finance Committee. *J Neur Sci* 1964; **1**: 88–9.

12 **Soetens A.** Report on the Participation of the Problem Commission of Neuro-anaesthesia in the Meeting of the Executive Committee of the World Federation of Neurosurgical Societies. *J Neur Sci* 1964; **1**: 96–7.

13 **Walton J.** The World Federation of Neurology. Chapter 20 (pp. 573–88) in *The Spice of Life. From Northumbria to World Neurology.* Royal Society of Medicine Services. London 1993.

14 **Matzke H.** Report on the Activities of the WFN Problem Commission of neuroradiology. *J Neur. Sci* 1964; **1**:394–6.

15 **Baker AB, Reesch JA, Loewenson RB:** Cerebral Atherosclerosis in European Populations: A Preliminary Report. *Stroke* 1973; **4**: 898–903.

16 **Van Bogaert.** Report on the Activities of the WFN Cerebrovascular Project (1961–63). *J Neur Sci* 1964; **1**: 98–103.

17 **Poser CM.** A Cooperative Effort in International Neurology. *World Neurol* 1960; **1**(1): 4–5.

18 **Glaser G.** Les cortico-stéroides ET l´ACTH dans les affections nerveuses. *World Neurol* 1960; **1**(1): 12–21.

19 **Walton J.** Die progressive. Muskeldystrophie—gegenwärtiger Forschungsstand. *World Neurol* 1960; **1**(2): 156–65.

20 **Refsum S.** Heredopathia atáctica polyneuritiformis. Reconsideración. *World Neurol* 1960; **1**(4): 334–47.

21 **Kurland L, Faro S, Siedler H.** Minamata Disease. The outbreak of a Neurologic disorder in Minamata, Japan, and its relationship to the ingestion of seafood contaminated by mercuric compounds. *World Neurol* 1960; **1**(5): 370–95.

22 **Pruzanski W, Altman R.** Encephalitis due to West Nile Fever virus. *World Neurol* 1962; **2**(6): 524–35.

23 **Geoffroy H, Slomic A, Benebadji M, Pascal P.** Myélo-polynévrites Tri-Crésyl Phospha-tées. *World Neurol* 1960; **1**(4): 294–315.

24 **Radermecker J.** Report on the activities of the Liaison Committee of the World Federa-tion of Neurology and the International Federation of EEG Societies (IFEEGS) in 1964. *J Neur Sci* 1965; **2**:581–2.

25 **Van Bogaert L.** Report of the WFN President Ludo van Bogaert. *J Neur Sci* 1966; **3**:96–105.

26 **Bailey P.** Report of Meeting of WFN Policy Committee (Vienna, 15 June 1963), and Report of the WFN Executive Committee Meeting. *J Neur Sci* 1964; **1**:91–6.

27 **Van Bogaert L.** World Federation of Neurology: Information. Meeting of the WFN Executive Committee, *J Neur Sci* 1965: **2**: 293–8.

28 **Van Bogaert L.** Presidential Report. WFN Executive Committee Meeting. *J Neur Sci* 1966; **3**:444–50.

29 **Bailey P.** Meeting of the WFN Executive Committee (El Escorial, Madrid, Spain, May 8–9, 1964). *J Neur Sci* 1965; **2**:293–6.

30 **Van Bogaert L.** Closing Remarks of President van Bogaert. *J Neur Sci* 1965; **2**:296–7.

31 **Van Bogaert L.** Minutes of the Meeting of the Secretaries of the WFN Problem Com-missions. (Institut Bunge, Berchem-Antwerp, 12 December 1964). *J Neur Sci* 19652: 575–6.

32 **Miller D.** Macdonald Critchley (1900–97) *J Med Biogr* 2006; **14**: 149.

33 **Rose FC.** Obituary. MacDonald Critchley (1900–1997) *World Neurol* 1997; **12**(4): 10.

34 **Rose FC.** Macdonald Critchley. In F Clifford Rose and WE Bynum Eds, *Historical Aspects of the Neurosciences.* Raven Press, New York 1982 , pp. ix–x.

35 **Critchley M.** *The Divine Banquet of the Brain and Other Essays.* Raven Press, New York 1979, pp. 178–82.

36 **Walton J.** The Spice of Life. From Northumbria to *World Neurol.* Chapter 20: The World Federation of Neurology. Royal Society of Medicine Services, London 1993.

37 **Critchley M.** World Federation of Neurology. President's Report. September 1969. *J Neurol Sci* 1970; **10**: 507–9.

38 **Critchley M.** World Federation of Neurology. President's Report 1973. *J Neurol Sci* 1974; **21**: 505–7.

39 **Bailey P.** Minutes Executive Committee Meeting. Vienna, 4 September 1965. *J Neurol Sci* 1966; **3**: 439–50.

40 **Critchley M.** Meeting of the Research Committee (formerly World Association of Neu-rological Commissions) Geneva, 1– 2 July 1966. *J Neurol Sci* 1967; **4**: 365–8.

41 **Miller H.** Minutes of the Executive Committee of the World Federation of Neurology. (Neurological Institute, New York, 25 June 1967). *J Neurol Sci* 1968; **6**: 386–9.

42 **Adeloye A, Ruberti R.** *The Pan African Association of Neurological Sciences (PAANS) The First Thirty Years 1972-2002.* Book Builders, Ibadan 2008.

43 **Nyberg-Hansen R.** Sigvald Refsum in memoriam–8 July. *World Neurol* 1991; **6**(4): 5–6.

44 **Walton J.** A personal postscript by Lord Walton of Detchant, President of the World Federation of Neurology. *World Neurol* 1991; **6**(4): 6.

45 **Olivarius B F.** Secretary-Treasurer General's Report 1975. *J Neurol Sci* 1976; **29**:429–32.

46 **Refsum S.** President's Report, Council of Delegates 1977. *J Neurol Sci* 1978; **36**:289–300.

47　**Walton J.** Editor-in-Chief's Report, Council of Delegates 1975. *J Neurol Sci* 1976; **29**:432–5.

48　**Walton J.** Newsletter of the Research Committee of the World Federation of Neurology. *J Neurol Sci* 1979; **40**: 197–201.

49　**World Federation of Neurology: Information.** Minutes of the meeting of the Executive Committee of the Research Group on Cerebral Vascular Disease (CVD) of the WFN. *J Neurol Sci* 1980; **46**: 255–6.

50　**Meeting of the Research Committee.** *J Neurol Sci* 1979; **43**: 483–9.

51　**The Statutes of the Research Committee of the World Federation of Neurology.** *J Neurol Sci* 1979; **43**: 490–3.

52　**Themes for Consideration by the Organizing Committee of the Next World Congress of Neurology in Japan in 1981.** *J Neurol Sci* 1979; **43**: 488–9.

53　**Oransky I, Richard L.** Masland. *Lancet* 2004; **363**(9409): 663.

54　**Lowenthal A.** Meeting of the Steering Committee of the World Federation of Neurology. *J Neur Sci* 1983; **58**:153–6.

55　**Juul Jensen P.** World Federation of Neurology: Council of Delegates. *J Neur Sci* 1982; **54**: 445–53.

56　**Toole JF.** World Federation of Neurology: Meeting of Council of Delegates Hamburg 1983. *J Neur Sci* 1984; **65**: 249–60.

57　**Bruyn G.** Report of the Finance Committee to the Steering Committee. *J Neur Sci* 1984; **65**: 259.

58　**Bruyn G.** Report of the WFN Finance Committee. *J Neur Sci* 1988; **85**: 98–9.

59　**Poeck K.** Minutes of the Meeting of the Steering Committee. *J Neur Sci* 1988; **85**: 97–8.

60　**Toole JF.** Minutes of the Council of Delegates Meeting. *J Neur Sci* 1988; **85**: 99–103.

61　**Walton J.** A message from the President. *World Neurol* 1989; **4**(3): 2.

62　**Toole JF.** Minutes of the Council of Delegates Meeting. *J Neur Sci* 1990; **97**: 326–32.

63　**Clifford Rose F.** Proposals for the Future Governance of the World Federation of Neurology. *World Neurol* 1996; **11**(3): 4.

64　**Blakesley A.** WFN Financial Report. *World Neurol* 1997; **12**(2): 4.

65　**Clifford Rose F.** Putting Advice into Action. *World Neurol* 1997; **12**(1): 1–4.

66　**Clifford Rose F.** Establishing a Permanent Secretariat. *World Neurol* 1997; **12**(2); 1–4.

67　**Clifford Rose F.** Reorganization of the Federation. *World Neurol* 1998; **13**(2); 1–3.

68　**Clifford Rose F.** Nine Successful Years of Growth and Change for the WFN. *World Neurol* 1999; **13**(4): 1–3.

69　**Godwin-Austen R.** Report of the Secretary-Treasurer General. *World Neurol* 1999; **14**(1): 8.

70　**Asbury AK.** Decade of the Brain. *World Neurol* 1990; **5**(1): 15.

71　**Nuwer MR, Lücking CH.** Wave Length and Action Potentials: History of the International Federation of Clinical Neurophysiology. *Clin Neurophysiol* 2010; **61** (Suppl).

72　**Roach ES, Bettermann K, Biller J.** *Toole's Cerebrovascular Disorders.* 6th ed. Cambridge University Press, Cambridge 2012.

73　**Toole JF.** WFN Strategic Planning for Next Millennium. *World Neurol* 1999; **14**(1): 1–6.

74　**Kimura J.** Report of the First Vice President. *World Neurol* 2001; **16**(1): 6–7.

75 **Toole JF.** XVIIth World Congress of Neurology, London, June 17–22, 2001. *World Neurol* 2001; **16**(3): 1–7.

76 **Toole JF.** Editorial. *World Neurol* 2001; **16**(4): 1–5.

77 Minutes of the Trustees' Meeting 14 December 2002, at the Medical Society of London.

78 Report on the WFN Structure and Function Committee about the management of WFN affairs (November 2003).

79 Minutes from the Annual General Meeting/Council of Delegates 5 September 2004.

80 Minutes from the WFN Trustees' Conference Call 15 March 2006.

81 **Spinney L.** A Neurologist Strikes a Nerve. *Intelligent Life* **17** April 2010.

82 **Shakir R.** Report of Secretary-Treasurer General. *World Neurol* 2007; **22**(1): 6.

83 **Platform Presentations of Presidential Nominees Sydney 2005.** *World Neurol* 2005; **20**(2): 7.

84 **World Health Organization.** *Neurological Disorders: Public Health Challenges.* WHO Press, Geneva 2006 (218 pp.).

85 **Aarli J.** World Federation of Neurology is growing. *World Neurol* 2007(3); **22**: 4–5.

Chapter 3

The World Federation of Neurology: Structure and Organization

Although the structure of the WFN had been modified since the organization was founded in 1957, it gradually became clear that the challenges of the modern world had surpassed the Federation's structural framework. The organization had grown considerably with increasing demands upon the Federation. The WFN had to face the challenges of a new age.

No one realized this better than John Walton, who was elected WFN President in 1989. His presidency became the most constructive modernization phase in the history of the WFN. The modernization lasted during the presidencies of Walton and Toole.

One of the most central steps of reorganization of the WFN was to establish corporate status for the WFN. Instead of a slow modernization process, the WFN decided during Walton's presidency to unwind the 'old', and establish the 'new' WFN. All WFN members were approached and involved in this process. For the last three years of Toole's presidency, the 'new' incorporated WFN co-existed alongside the 'old'. The meeting of the Council of Delegates in London on 17 June 2001 was an important historic event for the WFN because the 'old' organization was formally dissolved there.

The Companies Acts 1985 and 1989 (Memorandum and Articles of Association) describe the basic structure of the 'new' WFN, and are included here (Appendix 1). To understand the background of the new document, we will first see how the old WFN structure had developed over the years.

An archaic organization

Ludo van Bogaert had been the mover and shaker in the creation of the new federation. He had been sceptical about the club-like structure of neurology congresses before the Second World War:

> I was convinced that the old system of organization without constitutional statutes, under the control of well-known neurologists who were constantly elected and re-elected by their friends or by themselves, excluded the possibility of continuity and indispensable administrative responsibility. Such an organization was not truly

international in scope even though there existed the wonderful charm, familiarity and intimacy, which regrettably I have seen, disappear. In spite of the undeniable efficiency of such a system I felt that in view of the evolution of scientific and professional condition in our times, this type of organization was rapidly becoming archaic (1).

But van Bogaert was not alone. Two American neurologists, Houston Merritt and Pearce Bailey, were already familiar with the idea of a world neurological federation, which they had discussed at the meeting of the American Academy of Neurology (AAN) in Boston in April 1956. And while van Bogaert was not primarily a clinician, but an outstanding neuropathologist whose laboratory served as a magnet that attracted neuroscientists from all over the world, Merritt and Bailey were among the most respected and best clinical neurologists in the USA and knew clinical problems from the inside. In Boston, they had proposed the organization of a global neurology organization, to which the Academy offered its whole-hearted support.

A committee, consisting of van Bogaert, Merritt, Bailey, Critchley, Tournay, and Schaltenbrand, had drafted a constitution in both English and French. The proposal was discussed and accepted in Brussels in July 1957.

The most critical problems for the organization in 1957 were *the geographic factors, the language barriers,* and *the existing political situation* that might produce virtual scientific isolation. The new organization would have to implement international congresses of neurology and establish the Problem Commissions. This was the first step in organizing international research in neurology. Then came the establishment of regional neurological associations in other parts of the world (outside North America and Europe). But it was the Problem Commissions that took most of the time. In addition came economic problems because the income from annual dues in no way corresponded with the expenditure. These factors contributed to the first financial crisis.

Many decisions had to be taken by van Bogaert and Bailey. They could convene periodic Problem Commission meetings, while the WFN Executive Committee (later renamed the Council of Delegates) met only every second year. The regional organizations were not yet well developed. The economy of the Problem Commissions was problematic. There was no educational programme. There were considerable linguistic and financial problems, and the structure of the Federation had become archaic.

Meanwhile: what was the primary function of the WFN Executive Committee? Who should decide?

Did the WFN Executive Committee have any power?

The power of the Executive Committee (the Council of Delegates) is best illustrated when considering the discussion of the WFN Decentralization Plan. The

THE WORLD FEDERATION OF NEUROLOGY: STRUCTURE AND ORGANIZATION | **87**

WFN Policy Committee had approved the WFN Decentralization Plan at a meeting in Cologne in 1962. The WFN President, Ludo van Bogaert, and the Secretary-Treasurer General, Pearce Bailey, were both in favour of decentralization, but were also loyal to the decisions taken by the Executive Committee.

The plan concerned the decentralization of the administrative and geographical part of the Federation. An important element was the establishment of the regional organizations. Pearce Bailey called the national delegates from the American continent to a meeting in Lima, Peru, in 1963, where the first Pan-American Congress of Neurology took place. On behalf of most of the delegates, Professor Oscar Trelles (Peru) stated that decentralization would entail major expenses, and the actual and present state of the budget of the WFN could not support such a cost (2). Neither van Bogaert nor Bailey believed the WFN could survive without decentralization. As pointed out by Trelles during the discussion, regional decentralization might in future represent administrative advantages for the WFN, which is exactly what happened many years later with the formation of the regional neurological associations.

The WFN Executive Committee met at El Escorial, Madrid, in May 1964, and Bailey pointed out that the WFN decentralization process had already started and that the main question would be if it should be preplanned with a sense of direction. Van Bogaert was clear, 'I see in decentralization an undeniable necessity and one of great need', 'If you do not accept decentralization, I can promise you a collapse of the World Federation' (3). In a supplementary digest from the meeting, the report from the Committee on Decentralization, chaired by Graeme Robertson, was presented. There was a long discussion, and the voting showed 26 votes in favour of decentralization, with eight abstentions. At the Executive Committee Meeting the following year, in Vienna, van Bogaert concluded, not precisely defined, in his Presidential Report 'it seems to me – from a philosophical point of view – that it is neither indispensable nor fruitful to submerge individual continents in a universal totality where they run the risk of becoming ineffective or ignored' (4).

At the next meeting of the WFN Executive Committee, in New York in 1967, the new WFN President, Macdonald Critchley, stated that the earlier scheme for decentralization upon which a decision had been postponed for two years should be postponed indefinitely. This was unanimously approved (5).

So ended the long discussion on decentralization. The final result revealed that the power lay with the Council of Delegates.

The Council of Delegates

The Council of Delegates, previously named the WFN Executive Committee, was and still is the ruling body of the Federation. It consists of the national delegates of the national neurological associations. Theoretically, the Council of Delegates has the power to decide upon fundamental questions, but this is impractical for daily business because the meetings are so infrequent. In 1957, the Council of Delegates met only every second year. Even now, the Council of Delegates meets only once a year.

The WFN must hold an annual general meeting every year, which all member societies are entitled to attend. An authorized delegate, who is an individual member of the society, represents the member societies.

If it is clear that the authorized delegate of a member society is unable to be present, the Council of Delegates may appoint any member of that society or the authorized delegate of another member society to act on its behalf as its authorized delegate at that meeting (proxy). However, no authorized delegate can represent more than three member societies at any meeting. There is a quorum of a meeting of the Council of Delegates, if the number of authorized delegates personally present must be at least 15. A quorum of 15 can be obtained without much difficulty and the use of modern communications can facilitate meaningful contribution from those delegates not personally attending the meeting. If a delegate is appointed an Officer or Trustee, he/she ceases to be an authorized delegate from the date he or she starts to hold office. The appropriate member society then usually appoints another authorized delegate from that date.

The Policy Committee

It was important for van Bogaert and Bailey to have a small group of executive members, called the WFN Policy Committee, with intimate knowledge and understanding of the Federation. The Policy Committee was established in 1957, and was responsible for daily business without due consultation with the member societies.

During the formative period of the WFN and the first financial crisis, several situations occurred where the President, Ludo van Bogaert, and the Secretary-Treasurer General, Pearce Bailey, needed advice from the national delegates.

The members of the Policy Committee were the President, the Secretary-Treasurer General, the Treasurer and (later) the Secretary of the Research Committee, and the Editor-in-Chief of the *Journal of the Neurological Sciences*. The balance between the Policy Committee and the leadership group was uncomplicated. To some, the members were 'the usual suspects'.

What's in a name? The Steering Committee

It was decided in 1969 that because the names 'Policy Committee' and 'Executive Committee' had different meanings in different countries, these committees should in future be known as the *Steering Committee* and the *Council of Delegates*, respectively (6).

Since 1993, the President, the Secretary-Treasurer General, the First Vice President, and the Editor-in-Chief of the *Journal of the Neurological Sciences* have constituted the WFN Management Committee. Their function is to advise the Council of Delegates and the various Committees upon the issues of policy and day-to-day management (7).

Previously, the Council of Delegates met every second year, during the World Congress of Neurology, and once in the intervening years. It was clear that the meetings of the Council of Delegates should become annual, but the first regular annual meeting took place as late as 1999.

It soon became clear that the function of the new governance element had made the Steering Committee unnecessary. It first became the Long Range Planning Committee to emphasize its primary responsibility, but it was soon clear that one of the Trustees' main functions is long-range planning. The WFN Steering Committee was therefore disbanded when the 'new' WFN was organized in 2001.

The WFN Trustees

One major element of the new WFN is the appointment of Trustees. The Trustees are not the 'usual suspects' as was said about the old WFN leadership. When complete, the Trustees consist of the President, the First Vice President, the Secretary-Treasurer General, and three persons elected in accordance with the Articles of Association, and up to two co-opted persons. The Trustees are charity Trustees and have control of the Federation and its property and funds.

Since the ultimate power is vested in the Council of Delegates, the Trustees may exercise any powers of the Federation which are not reserved to the Council of Delegates. The Trustees can make Rules consistent with the Memorandum, and Articles of Association to govern proceedings at meetings of the Council of Delegates. The Trustees can also make Rules consistent with these Articles to govern proceedings at their meetings and at meetings of committees.

The Trustees can delegate functions to for example a Finance Committee and the proceedings of that committee must be reported promptly to the Trustees.

The Committees of the WFN

The WFN has several committees, which have had different functions and have been created in different phases of the organization's history. Some of them have been disbanded. The present WFN committees (2011) are the Africa Initiative, the (Applied) Research Committee, the Asia Initiative, the WFN Congress Supervisory Committee, the Constitution & Bye-laws Committee, the Education Committee, the Evaluation and Accreditation Committee, the Finance Committee, the Fund-Raising Committee, the Latin America Initiative, the Membership Committee, the Nominating Committee, the Public Awareness & Action Committee, and the Publications Committee.

The Constitution & Bye-laws Committee has been retained because it was felt that the Memorandum and Articles of Association might require more detailed rules and regulations than those appropriate for former committees. This Committee with Jun Kimura as chair decided to tackle this revision in two stages. The first stage consisted of adding all the changes already approved by the COD after the 1990 Indian Congress (XV-WCN), when the last version of the Constitution & Bye-laws was produced.

The second stage was to make further radical modifications to ensure that all practices were fully compatible with the Articles of Association once the WFN was incorporated under UK law as a company limited by guarantee. Gathering the information for the first step proved to be easier said than done, primarily because Kimura had to locate the specific wording of the modifications that were scattered in different documents over the span of ten years. Recent personnel changes within the organization and the relocation of the Secretariat also made it difficult to pinpoint the exact source of information. With help from the members of the Executive Committee and Keith Newton at the London Office, however, all the papers pertinent to the revision were collected. The chair of the committee in 2011 was Michael Donaghy (UK).

The Applied Research Committee, Constitution & Bye-laws Committee, the Finance Committee, the Membership Committee, the Nominating Committee and the Publications Committee are the oldest committees of the Federation. The Africa Initiative, the Asia Initiative, and the Latin America Initiative are discussed in Chapter 6. WFN Committees that were initiated after 2007 are not discussed here.

The Finances of the WFN

The Office of the WFN Secretary-Treasurer General

The office of the WFN Secretary-Treasurer General has always been important, in particular during financial crises. The Secretary-Treasurer General has close contact with and was for a long time *ex officio* the chairman of the Finance Committee.

Pearce Bailey was the first WFN Secretary-Treasurer General. Before that, he had been the Director of the NINDB, to which he was appointed in 1951.

THE WORLD FEDERATION OF NEUROLOGY: STRUCTURE AND ORGANIZATION | **91**

During the first years of its existence, the economy of the WFN was totally dependent upon the NINDB. Bailey was, together with van Bogaert, in office during the first eight years. He oversaw the early development and took care to prepare the Federation for the new situation that would occur when the WFN would have to depend completely upon its own annual dues and other forms of income.

Pearce Bailey and Ludo van Bogaert both believed that decentralization would be crucial for the economy. Decentralization was never implemented, and the income from the annual dues was erratic. The next Secretary-Treasurer General was Henry Miller. Like Bailey, he was also the chairman of the Finance Committee. Miller had to face a new financial situation, and at the first meeting of the Council of Delegates, in New York in 1967, when he had been in office for only two years, expenditure had exceeded income 'to some extent', so that it was necessary to draw on capital. At the same time, some of the expenditure was non-recurring, arising as it did from the transfer of the secretariat from Antwerp to London. Although the Executive Committee approved the balance sheet, they concluded that chartered accountants should in future audit it.

It became clear at the New York meeting in 1967 that the finances of the then new Research Committee (see later) would represent a separate responsibility, and that the Secretary-Treasurer of the Research Committee would have to present their accounts in time to incorporate them with the annual balance sheet of the WFN. Henry Miller realized that it would be difficult to delineate the expenses of the various Research Groups, and that the reorganized Committee would be much easier to control than the conglomerate of the old Problem Commissions.

Two years later, in New York in 1969, the audited statement of accounts was in balance and was approved unanimously. The Finance Committee had decided that, at the discretion of the President and the Secretary-Treasurer General, grants might be made from the WFN's capital sum of money in special circumstances. In Barcelona in 1973, when Refsum's administration took over, there was still a capital sum for Henry Miller to hand over to his successor as Secretary-Treasurer General, Bent de Fine Olivarius, although the running costs of the WFN had been increasing.

The winter of our discontent

Two years later, in Amsterdam in 1975, Olivarius was unable to present an audited balance sheet. He took the opportunity to explain that the daily work as Secretary-Treasurer was superimposed upon his duties as head of a very active and busy department, extensive undergraduate and postgraduate teaching, scientific work, and many duties in his Faculty of Medicine (8). It had been difficult to transfer the WFN funds from England to Denmark, and £8,000 was only transferred in June 1974. He also had the approval of the Finance Committee to have the fiscal year run from June to June, and pointed out that the administration costs had never been as low in the history of the WFN.

When the Council of Delegates next met, in Amsterdam in 1977, Olivarius was unable to attend owing to illness, and Palle Juul-Jensen, also of Aarhus, Denmark, was appointed Assistant Secretary. This required acceptance by the Council, which elected him Acting Secretary-Treasurer General (9). Juul-Jensen was also unable to present accounts at the meeting, because Olivarius had requested his assistance only six days previously. Juul-Jensen could therefore say nothing about the financial situation, except that the present funds had been reduced by almost 50% since 1973. If this continued, the WFN would be without money by 1981.

Events had shown that revision of the WFN Constitution & Bye-laws had become urgent. The revised version was approved at the meeting of the Council of Delegates in Kyoto in 1979. In future, the Secretary-Treasurer General would be required to present a true balance of the Federation's financial status at the end of each fiscal year. The WFN Finance Committee would initiate an annual review of the financial record of the Federation and would provide for the auditing of the books of the Secretary-Treasurer annually.

In Kyoto in 1981, the WFN financial situation remained weak, although it improved considerably under Juul-Jensen's leadership. Pierre Dreyfus (USA) was first elected Secretary-Treasurer General with Palle Juul-Jensen as Joint Secretary-Treasurer General. After some time, Dreyfus informed the WFN that he had to decline the position and James Toole was appointed. He had at his side the former Secretary-Treasurer General Palle Juul-Jensen.

At the Council of Delegates in Hamburg 1983, Toole informed the delegates that the WFN communication network had been disappointing. Fortunately, the 12th World Congress of Neurology in Kyoto had been a success and brought the WFN a sum of DM18,000.

Toole managed the budget situation very carefully and had close collaboration with the chairman of the WFN Finance Committee (and also the Editor-in-Chief of the *Journal of the Neurological Sciences*), George Bruyn. At the Council of Delegates in Hamburg 1985, the importance of loans made by the WFN to each World Congress being repaid in full at an early stage was also pointed out.

The financial situation of the WFN had become chaotic during Refsum's presidency, because of the Secretary-Treasurer General's illness. The changes to the constitution, which had been accomplished in 1979, were implemented, and the financial administration of the WFN changed considerably during

Masland's presidency. The role of chairman of the WFN Finance Committee became much more important, and the Secretary-Treasurer General was now able to oversee the structure and organization of the Federation.

At the Council of Delegates in Hamburg, George Bruyn was re-elected chairman of the Finance Committee while Sir John Walton became chairman of the Constitution & Bye-laws Committee. Palle Juul-Jensen became chairman of the Steering Committee, a position that Klaus Poeck (Germany) soon took over.

The WFN Finance Committee

> But Central Bankers are not paid, Mr. President, to look on the bright side of things. We are paid to worry, to worry about what might go wrong and to anticipate the clouds coming over the horizon.
> (*Mr Eddie George, the British Central Bank Bankers Club, London, 2004*)

Both Pearce Bailey and Henry Miller had each been WFN Secretary-Treasurer General and chairman of the Finance Committee. They had presented formal reports on the WFN sources of income, expenditures, and balances. During the period 1961–1963, total funds were $109,407.12. This amount had been stable as long as the NINDB grants arrived. Bailey was a safe hand with the organization's finances, and he knew the NINDB and WFN well. However, the flow of US seed money had come to an end.

The first financial crisis of the WFN arose when the economic support from the NINDB disappeared, and was soon aggravated because many member societies did not pay the annual dues. In his report to the WFN Executive Committee in Vienna in 1965, van Bogaert explained that the WFN was now for the first time on its own financially, and he recommended 'adoption and promulgation of the Decentralization Plan in order to provide for a greater division of labour in the financing of the WFN and for a more world-wide participation in its programs' (4). In van Bogaert's mind, the Decentralization Plan included the possibility of obtaining financial support from each region. But the society chose another way.

Henry Miller was elected Secretary-Treasurer General in Vienna in 1965. Together with David Klein, the Secretary-Treasurer General of the (new) Research Committee, they controlled the administrative expenses.

New problems arose in 1973. Palle Juul-Jensen was Acting Secretary-Treasurer General, George W. Bruyn (the Netherlands), J.M. Espadaler Medina (Spain), and Olle Thage (Denmark) became new members of the WFN Finance Committee.

George W. Bruyn was the new chairman of the Finance Committee. The interplay between the office of the Secretary-Treasurer and the Finance

94 | THE HISTORY OF THE WORLD FEDERATION OF NEUROLOGY

Committee was now better organized. Although the financial situation approached crisis in the late 1980s, Bruyn anticipated clouds coming over the horizon in due time, and the necessary precautions were taken to save the Federation.

Masland's presidency was the first time that the Chairman of the WFN Finance Committee presented a full report to the Council of Delegates. George Bruyn, who had just been appointed Chairman, reported that expenses, if the Finance Committee accepted the proposed budget, would exceed income by US$1,025. The Finance Committee therefore decided to reduce the budget to US$12,500, and it was this sum that would be transferred to the 13th World Congress of Neurology, as an interest-free loan (10–12). The problem of finance had again reared its ugly head.

When the WFN administration was reorganized during Walton's presidency, it was decided that the Finance Committee should consist of three or more individuals, each of whom must be an individual member of a National Neurological Society. The Trustees should appoint them, and at least one of them should be a Trustee.

Robert Daroff had been a member of the Finance Committee from 1985, and he was the Chairman during the critical reconstruction period 1990–2001 and contributed strongly to the successful result.

WFN annual dues

From the beginning, the annual member society dues were $1 per member of each constituent society. From the beginning, both the AAN and the American Neurological Association paid regularly. The AAN paid a total of much more than any other single member society and the American Neurological Association also paid its dues regularly. The AAN is still the main contributor because it has the greatest number of active members.

In 1963, the WFN Executive Committee voted to increase the dues to $2, and many societies paid the increased figure. Others did not. Some societies paid promptly and regularly, others were late and intermittent, and some were delinquent. A few societies never paid any dues. For 1964, societies from 12 countries were delinquent. Accordingly, payments were not made regularly. Bailey and van Bogaert had regarded the WFN decentralization proposal as the only way to save the organization. But the next administration decided to postpone it, and the annual dues were not formally raised until the second part of Macdonald Critchley's presidency, when the Council of Delegates unanimously voted to increase the annual membership fee to $2 per individual member of each society.

Bailey had pointed out at the meeting of the WFN Executive Committee at El Escorial in May 1964, that if the annual dues were increased from $1 to $2 per active member—and if these payments were made regularly—one could estimate an annual income from these funds after 1965 of approximately $8,000 per annum, which would permit financial support of a Central Secretariat with a secretarial staff, but would not allow for any extensive programming, travel, or support of Problem Commissions. For this purpose, it would be essential to develop a new methodology of fund-raising and/or new sources of support. The only proposal thus far to meet this emergency was the WFN decentralization proposal.

If payment of annual dues was related to the capacity for the organization of regional groups, Bailey thought the easiest task would belong to the Greater European Association, which had paid total dues to the amount of $10,233, followed by the Greater American with $6,585, and finally the Asian-Oceanian with $946.

In his President's Report in New York in 1969, Macdonald Critchley was clear:

> Nowadays the financial resources of the Federation are—to put it mildly—minimal. The income received each year from each of the national societies just—only just— meets the day to day expenses entailed in an extensive world-wide correspondence. Unfortunately, it is no longer possible to meet the expenses of travel, and regrettably it is no longer feasible to give financial support to secretariat and delegates who put in such hard work in connection with the various Research Groups, symposia, etc. (7).

Due to insufficient information from the WFN, relatively few national societies had paid their annual subscription from 1974 onwards. The WFN funds had therefore been just adequate to cover secretarial and other minor administrative costs. Sigvald Refsum as President, and Palle Juul-Jensen as Acting Secretary-Treasurer General now decided to provide exact information to the secretariats of national societies about the delinquent societies. Newsletters were sent out in March 1978, October 1978, and April 1979. As a result, a number of societies paid the dues, and the financial situation of the WFN improved. Juul-Jensen was, however, still unable to finalize the accounts for the last years of his predecessor. In 1983, it was discussed whether societies that had not paid the annual dues should lose WFN membership. This threat was never implemented, but societies that had not paid annual dues would not be able to vote during the Council of Delegates.

Income from the WFN Congresses

The WFN income increased from the 1990s onwards. The most important financial element in this process was the preliminary interest-free grant to the host society responsible for each World Congress of Neurology. It was agreed in Hamburg during the world congress in 1985 that the WFN would be given a proportion of the profits made by that congress. The congress in New Delhi in 1989 did generate a substantial profit, but under Indian government regulations, the money could not be transferred to WFN central funds but had to stay in India to support activities sponsored by the Federation in that country.

The next world congress took place in Vancouver, Canada, in 1993, and it was agreed that 50% of the profits should be retained by the host society, and 50% transferred to the WFN in return for the WFN administrative costs involved in planning the congress and programme in collaboration with its Research Committee.

The WFN income also increased because of the increase in annual dues from an increased number of member societies and the royalties from its scientific journals. Developments in the neurosciences had increased and new and effective drugs were available. As a consequence, registration fees, advertisements, exhibit hall rentals, and sponsorships were new sources of income.

During the latter part of the 1990s, the WFN gradually developed into a financially successful organization.

The Nominating Committee

The function of the Nominating Committee is to solicit nominations for the offices of the President, the Vice President, and the Officers.

The Trustees form the Nominating Committee. The number of persons in the Nominating Committee is small (four or five), and they are required to present their report to the Secretary-Treasurer General in time for the meeting of the Council of Delegates. The Secretary-Treasurer General then presents the report, which is usually approved by unanimous consent. That means that the national delegates for all practical purposes have accepted the proposed candidates for the positions. This routine has changed gradually over the years.

The first challenge for the Nominating Committee came when President Ludo van Bogaert retired in 1965. In Vienna in 1965, the Chairman of the Nominating Committee, Helmuth Tschabitscher (Vienna) presented the following list of candidates: President Macdonald Critchley, Vice Presidents Graeme Robertson (Australia), S. Sarkisov (Moscow), Francois Thiébaut (Strasbourg), and Oscar Trelles (Lima), and as Secretary-Treasurer General Henry Miller. The President and Vice Presidents were to serve for a period of four years. The President could be and was re-elected, but the Vice Presidents could not.

The election of Vice Presidents was informally regarded as an election of Regional Vice Presidents. When it came to the post-election facts, geographical considerations were not dominant. In addition, as Europe was split by the Iron Curtain, it effectively served as two different regions.

Graeme Robertson (Australia) was elected President of the Nominating Committee at the Congress in Vienna in 1965. In New York in 1969, the Nominating Committee recommended the following for the election of officers for a term of four years: President: Macdonald Critchley. Editor of the *Journal of the Neurological Sciences*: John N. Walton. Regional Vice Presidents: Eddie Bharucha (India), E. Herman (Poland), Richard Masland (USA), Georg Schaltenbrand (Germany), and Velasco-Suarez (Mexico). The Executive Committee approved the recommendations unanimously.

In Barcelona in 1973, the candidates of the Nominating Committee were for the presidency: Sigvald Refsum. John Walton was re-elected Editor of the *Journal of the Neurological Sciences*. Vice Presidents: J. Game (Melbourne), G. Poech (Buenos Aires), J. Cernacek (Czechoslovakia), F. McNaughton (Montreal), and Eberhard Bay (Düsseldorf). The Council of Delegates endorsed the recommendations. Sigvald Refsum proposed Professor Bent de Fine Olivarius (Denmark) as the Secretary-Treasurer General, which was approved.

Alternative candidates for the WFN presidency

The first time alternative names appeared as candidates for the presidency was at the election in New Delhi in 1989. This did not imply that there were no alternative candidates before that time. In 1981, Richard Masland was unanimously elected President. Another distinguished US neurologist, Raymond Adams, was mentioned, but his name was withdrawn before the election (13).

At the 1989 elections, the Chairman of the Nominating Committee, Theodore Munsat, first presented its proposal to the Steering Committee. The Nominating Committee consisted of Theodore Munsat (Chairman), Antonio Spina-Franca (Brazil), Eijiro Satoyoshi (Japan), and J.G. McLeod (Australia). The WFN President, Richard Masland, presented the slate to the Council of Delegates and proposed that it should be approved. At the meeting of the Council of Delegates, however, it was requested that they be allowed to make additional nominations at their second meeting three days later. At the second meeting, John Walton, who was the Nominating Committee candidate, was elected by 32 votes cast in his favour with 17 votes for the alternative candidate, George Bruyn. Frank Clifford Rose was elected Secretary-Treasurer General and Klaus Poeck First Vice President.

There were eighth candidates for the five Vice President positions, and Arthur Asbury (USA), Ben Hamida (Tunisia), Alberto Portera-Sanchez (Spain),

98 | THE HISTORY OF THE WORLD FEDERATION OF NEUROLOGY

James Lance (Australia), and Noshir Wadia (India) were elected. This was democracy in operation.

The Officers of the Steering Committee and Finance Committee were also elected, as was the position of Editor of the *Journal of the Neurological Sciences*, and James Toole was elected by unanimous vote.

In 1993, the Nominating Committee proposed Walton, Rose, Poeck, and Toole for the same positions, which they had held for the last four years, and they were accepted unanimously. Henry J. Barnett (Canada), Armand Lowenthal (Belgium), P. Pinelli (Italy), A. Rascol (France), and Eijiro Satoyoshi (Japan) were elected Regional Vice Presidents. The Officers of the Steering Committee and the Finance Committee were also elected. No other nominations were put forward to the Congress.

It was decided at the Council of Delegates in Buenos Aires in 1995 that from 1997 on, the WFN President would hold his post for four years only, with no re-election. It was also decided that there would be a new post of Senior Vice President, separate from Chairman of the Research Committee, who would be elected by the Research Committee.

Recommendations for WFN elections

The WFN Nominating Committee chaired by Professor Eero Hokkanen (Finland) held formal meetings in Buenos Aires in 1995 and in Helsinki in 1996. These meetings were preceded by a comprehensive survey of the opinions of national societies and formal proposals made by national societies and national delegates and merit rating carried out by the chairman and the members of the committee (14).

In Buenos Aires in 1997, there were five candidates for the WFN presidency, namely Jagjit Chopra, Franz Gerstenbrand, James Lance, Klaus Poeck, and James F. Toole. There were also five candidates for the position of First Vice President: Antonio Culebras, Franz Gerstenbrand, Jun Kimura, F. Rubio Donnadieu, and James F. Toole. James Toole was elected WFN President, and Jun Kimura First Vice President. The former Chairman of the Research Committee was not included in the nomination process (15).

In London in 2001, there were two candidates for the presidency, First Vice President Jun Kimura, and Donald Paty (Canada). For the first time, their election addresses were published in *World Neurology* in addition to being presented at the election (16). There were also two candidates for First Vice President, Johan Aarli (Norway) and Roberto Sica (Argentina). At the elections in June 2001, Jun Kimura was elected WFN President, and Johan Aarli First Vice President.

The election procedures of the WFN, as they appeared after the London congress, had undergone a revolution. There were ten candidates for three vacancies for the new positions of Elected Trustee. Julien Bogousslavsky (Switzerland), William Carroll (Australia) and Roberto Sica (Argentina) were elected.

The candidates for the election at the World Congress in Sydney in 2005 were First Vice President Johan Aarli, Jagjit Chopra (India), Wolf-Dieter Heiss (Germany), and Roger Rosenberg (USA). There were two candidates for First Vice President, Vladimir Hachinski (Canada) and Theodore Munsat (USA). There were three candidates for the position of elected Trustee, Marianne De Visser (Netherlands), Michael Donaghy (UK), and Werner Hacke (Germany). Johan Aarli was elected WFN President, and Vladimir Hachinski First Vice President. Marianne De Visser was re-elected Trustee (17). For the first time, the platform presentations of the First Vice Presidential Nominees were also published in *World Neurology*, in addition to those of the four Nominees for the presidency (17,18).

According to the WFN constitution, the WFN Secretary-Treasurer General will be elected one year later than the election of the WFN Officers. This is to provide a suitable overlap between two subsequent administrations. Julien Bogousslavsky (Switzerland) had already been elected as Trustee designated to take over as the new Secretary-Treasurer General at the end of 2006, one year after Aarli had been elected WFN President. Due to unforeseen events in May 2006, Bogousslavsky had to resign from his position as a Trustee, and Raad Shakir was elected WFN Secretary-Treasurer General at the Council of Delegates in Glasgow in 2006 (19).

The 2006 Council of Delegates meeting took place in Glasgow during the annual EFNS Congress. Werner Hacke and Ryuji Kaji were elected Trustees.

The 2007 Council of Delegates met in Brussels during the EFNS Congress, which was also the WFN Silver Jubilee. The 2008 Council of Delegates met in New Delhi during the Asian Oceanian Congress, and then in 2009 in Bangkok during the World Congress, illustrating the globality of the Federation.

There were two nominees for the WFN presidency at the elections at the World Congress in Bangkok, Thailand, in 2009, Vladimir Hachinski and Jagjit Chopra, and three for the position as First Vice President, Leontino Batttistin (Italy), William Carroll (Australia), and Werner Hacke (Germany) (20). Werner Hacke was elected.

New guidelines for the Nominating Committee

According to the new constitution of 2001, the Nominating Committee is appointed by, and functions directly under, the President of the WFN, and is independent of the Secretariat. Its effective period is four years, but this was reduced to two years in 2011. The present Chairman is Dr Donald Silberberg, Philadelphia.

The present guidelines for the Nominating Committee are:

1 To solicit, by mail and other forms of communication, nominations for the offices of Trustee and Officer as defined in the 'Memorandum and Articles of Association of the WFN', at least one-and-a-half years before the appropriate AGM.

2 To evaluate the initial list of nominations sent to the Nominating Committee and scrutinize each nominee's stature, contributions, and commitment to the growth and development of the WFN.

3 To give due consideration to geography and gender in evaluating nominations and, if these considerations are lacking, supplement them by identifying appropriate candidates from the WFN database.

4 To request support of each nominee from his or her national neurological organization in identifying and verifying potential candidates for short listing.

5 To send the agreed list of nominees for Trustee and Officer, which may or may not be ranked, to the Secretariat in London in time for publication, including in the winter issue of *World Neurology* and the *Journal of Neurological Sciences* at least six months before the AGM for voting by WFN Delegates.

6 To add to that list all further nominations supported by the signatures of five (5) or more authorized Delegates for the offices of Trustee and Officer that are received by the Secretariat at least 30 days prior to the AGM.

The main function of the WFN Nominating Committee is to present a list with the number of candidates needed to fill the vacant positions. These positions are the President, the first Vice President, the Secretary-Treasurer General, and when needed, a candidate for the position of the Editorship of the *Journal of the Neurological Sciences* (21).

The Continuing Education Committee

The Education Committee is of relatively recent origin. It first materialized as a Research Group during the productive period of new thinking and reconstruction of the WFN during the 1990s. During Masland's presidency (1981–1989), Professor L.P.M. van der Lugt (Limburg, the Netherlands) had proposed to the WFN delegates the formation of a new Research Group for Neurological Education. The group was formed in 1983, and van der Lugt was its first Secretary (22). He presented a programme for the new Research Group. The report

THE WORLD FEDERATION OF NEUROLOGY: STRUCTURE AND ORGANIZATION | **101**

revealed uncertainty about the range of needs for development of a core curriculum in neurological education, and it was suggested that there be a fact-
finding survey to determine what a neurologist is, or should be. In some
countries, there were no standards and no examinations, while the requirements were excessively rigid in other countries. The need for knowledge of the
nervous system by non-neurologists was regarded overwhelming and might in
developing countries even be greater than for neurologists.

Later, the Research Group also sponsored the journal *Current Opinions in
Neurology and Neurosurgery*, and received in return an annual sum from the
publishers; 10% of that sum came to the WFN.

Neurological Education and the Research Group on Delivery of Neurological Services

Since there was no nomination to the Management Committee for a chairman,
John Walton asked Professor Barrows (Ill, USA) to take over. He was followed
by Jock Murray (Halifax, Nova Scotia) in 1986 and Mathew Menken in 1989.
When Menken (MA, USA) was the Secretary of the group, collaboration with
the Research Group on Delivery of Neurological Services was initiated. Together, they organized a seminar on Neurology in Developing Countries during the
annual AAN meeting in Miami, USA, in 1990 (23–25). Professor B.S. Singhal
(India) and colleagues organized a meeting on Neurological Education in Asia
and Oceania, illustrating the global importance of the issue (22). This was also
reflected in the resolution on neurological education presented at the 1st International Research Group on Delivery of Neurological Services Conference
'Neurology Update 2000' in New Delhi in 1994 (26). In 1993, the name of the
group was changed to Research Group on Medical Education, illustrating that
education in neurology is part of medical education.

The issue of neurological education was becoming more and more important,
and was discussed at the planning meeting for the World Congress of Neurology in Buenos Aires in 1995, when Professor Klaus Poeck, First Vice President
and Chairman of the Research Committee, presented practical and technical
problems associated with the certifying process for specialists in neurology and
the use of CME credits (27). Meanwhile, the AAN, the Royal College of Physicians in London as well as appropriate authorities in a number of other countries had accepted attendance of WFN members at WFN symposia and
congresses for CME accreditation.

Neurological Education and the WFN Research Committee

At the World Congress of Neurology in Vancouver, 1993, the Council of Delegates had established ad hoc Continuing Education and Public Relations

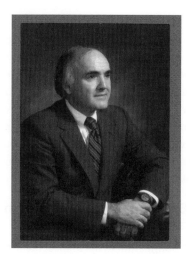

Fig. 3.1 Ted Munsat, Chairman of the Education Committee.

Courtesy of Ted Munsat.

Committees. Terms of reference were presented at the World Congress in Buenos Aires.

In Buenos Aires in 1997, Theodore Munsat (Figure 3.1) was elected as Chairman of the Research Committee and he also became Chairman of the WFN Education Committee. A major change in WFN educational activities came about when James Toole took office. The Strategic Planning Meeting held in St Albans (see earlier) was important. In 2001, Munsat became co-opted Chair of the WFN Education Committee while Professor Roger Rosenberg became Chair of the WFN Research Committee.

Munsat resigned as Chair of the Research Committee to concentrate on education. With his background as past AAN President and special insight and experience in continuing education in neurology, he initiated a series of pilot studies using the AAN programme *Continuum: Lifelong Learning in Neurology* (27).

During the next 10 years the WFN Education Committee and its activities grew. Early in the programme development it became clear that although education was well covered in Europe, by the EFNS and ENS, and in North America, by the AAN, there was a wide gap in services for underdeveloped and developing countries. Thus, the major thrust of the work was in that direction, and it was focused upon CME.

Munsat started three important initiatives in neurology education. The core educational programme has been the Continuum study group programme, which has involved 43 developing countries and about 8,500 individuals. Over the ten years of its existence, six-monthly reports have been provided to the Secretariat. The WFN *Seminars in Clinical Neurology*, edited by Pete Engel, is a series of texts established to provide authoritative information on neurological practice for the developing world.

The Committee also helped establish new neurology training programmes. The first was established in Honduras by Marco Medina and approved by the University of Honduras Educational Council. It developed into a comprehensive training programme, which has since been applied as a model in other parts of the world. The results have since been published in WFN reports and publications and the journal *Neurology*.

The third initiative is Education of Non-neurologists in Developing Countries, chaired by Gretchen L. Birbeck. She has developed, tested, and published online the programme 'Where There is No Neurologist: A Manual for Paramedicals in Developing Countries'.

The WFN Membership Committee

Twenty-six delegates from 21 countries were present at the WFN's birth in 1957. Fifty years later, the number had increased to 113.

Any national society of neurologists with more than five members may apply for membership of the WFN and can nominate a delegate to the Council of Delegates. The WFN Membership Committee reviews each letter of application and the credentials of the society and presents its advice to the Council of Delegates. In 2006, the Council of Delegates expressed the view that the WFN should be inclusive rather than exclusive in accepting membership applications.

For many years, few individual African countries had established national neurological societies. The PAANS, which is a supranational organization, had no voting rights. The Nigerian Society was formed in 1966, and new societies emerged in the subsequent years. There are obvious advantages of membership, in particular for developing countries, which clearly benefit from the educational programmes, and the Membership Committee therefore extended invitations to neurologists of non-member countries.

With the Chinese Neurological Society joining in 2007, the World Federation of Neurology has for the first time become a true global organization.

The WFN Publications Committee

The Publications Committee oversees and evaluates the WFN-sponsored journals and makes recommendations concerning the Editors. The two major WFN publications are the *Journal of the Neurological Sciences* and *World Neurology*.

In 1987, the WFN finances had reached a low level, and the WFN was also charged with obtaining resources from WFN-sponsored journals. The WFN Finance Committee recommended that a WFN Publications Subcommittee be formed and was chaired by Professor Robert Daroff, the chair of the Publications Committee 1987–2001.

The subcommittee started by scrutinizing the contracts of the *Journal of the Neurological Sciences*, *Journal of Neuroimmunology*, *Acta Neuropathologica*, and the new *World Neurology* newsletter. The annual contribution from the WFN concerning *Acta Neuropathologica* had ceased. The publisher did not regard the *Journal of Neuroimmunology* as being sponsored by the WFN. The contract with Raven Press concerning *World Neurology* was terminated on 31 December 1988 and efforts to obtain another publisher continued. The final agreement with Elsevier concerning the *Journal of the Neurological Sciences* had been agreed and signed.

The ownership of the copyright of the *Journal of the Neurological Sciences* belongs to Elsevier. Royalties were set at 10% of the net receipts. Renewal of the contract was 'automatic' unless there was a demonstrated breach on the part of the publisher. The new proposed contract put the emphasis on electronic publishing and dissemination. Elsevier has proposed an increase in royalties for the WFN as well as an increase in the Editorial Office budget.

World Neurology was for a long time produced and published in India and financed in part through a grant from the Japan Foundation for Neuroscience and Mental Health.

Over the years, WFN publications related to education, such as *Seminars in Clinical Neurology*, were organized through the WFN Publications Committee. The WFN website has its own Editor, but is also a part of the mandate of the Publications Committee. Professor Christopher Kennard (Oxford) is the present Chair. (2011)

The Public Relations and WHO Liaison Committee

At the Vancouver congress in 1993, President John Walton established a WFN Public Relations Committee with Professor Donald Paty as Chairman. Due to Professor Paty's health problems, Johan Aarli was invited by John Walton to take over as the new Chairman. Aarli included WHO Liaison Committee matters as its main function, and much of the Committee's work became focused on the effect of the collaboration between the WFN and the WHO, as exemplified by the reports on the Neurology Atlas, and Neurological Disorders. It then became more natural that this work became part of the Africa Initiative more than of a WFN Committee.

World Neurology Foundation

Professor James Toole founded the World Neurology Foundation (WNFo) in 1999 while he was the President of the WFN. He wrote in his Annual Report of the President for 1999:

THE WORLD FEDERATION OF NEUROLOGY: STRUCTURE AND ORGANIZATION | **105**

I have formed a World Federation of Neurology Foundation in the United States to take advantage of U.S. tax laws which encourage charitable donations. For those who would like such opportunities, this is a marvelous way to help neurology research and education worldwide (28).

Toole had discussed the project with the WFN Management Committee, which then consisted of President Toole, First Vice President Jun Kimura, Chairman of the Research Committee Theodore L. Munsat, and the Secretary-Treasurer General Frank Clifford Rose (succeeded by Richard Godwin-Austen as new Secretary-Treasurer General) (29,30). The Management Committee decided to form a charitable foundation exempted from taxes by the Internal Revenue Service in the United States (31).

The name of the foundation has changed during its existence. The name on the official letterhead on a letter dated 21 August 2000, is 'World Neurology Foundation (Devoted to education and research in association with the World Federation of Neurology, the World Health Organization, and 94 national societies and patient organizations)'. However, Toole convened the first meeting and conference call at the 'World Neurology Research and Education Foundation' at Chandos Street, London, 19 September 2000. He reported that a 501-C3 tax-exempt organization had now been obtained (29). It was made clear that the WFN and the Foundation are independent organizations that make their decisions independently of each other. The composition of the Board and its bye-laws and guidelines were discussed, and it was decided that the office of the Foundation would be in Winston-Salem and that Ms Dianne C. Vernon would continue to provide financial and secretarial assistance for the Foundation and the Board Members as the secretary-treasurer.

Funding of Endowed Lectureships is an important part of the Foundation's activities, and in March, 2001, the Masland Lectureship had collected $43,000 with pledges of $7,000 for the required $50,000, and the Yahr Lectureship $82,550 with pledges of $17,450 for the goal of $100,000. So far, the WNFo had sponsored named lectures at the World Congresses in Sydney (2005) and Bangkok. (2009) The matter of a 20% overhead for the Foundation was to be discussed. During Culebras' tenure, the WNFo received two endowments totalling $100,000 to the Singhal fund and the Eddie & Piloo Bharucha fund, to sponsor lectureships at the World Congress of Neurology.

The composition of the Board was changed in 2001 when Jun Kimura resigned when he became WFN President and Ted Munsat when he became head of the WFN Continuing Education Committee. Antonio Culebras (USA) and Jock Murray from Nova Scotia had been invited to join. Amos Korczyn (Israel) had previously been invited for WNFo conference calls.

The name WFN Research & Education Foundation was still the letterhead for the conference call on 11 June 2003, but it was agreed that fund-raising had not been successful for the Education Committee, and that the WFN Research Foundation and the Education Committee must work together. From 2003 on, the term World Neurology Foundation was used. Carrie Becker had previously worked together with Munsat for the WFN Education Committee on a WFN contract.

In an e-mail dated 4 October 2001, Toole commented upon the apparent duplication of the mission and responsibilities of the Research Committee for Continuing Education and the WFN research and education foundation, and was sceptical about fund-raising by the Education Committee (31).

The Board at this meeting consisted of James Toole, Richard Godwin-Austen, Richard Janeway, Antonio Culebras, Keith Newton, and Dianne Vernon. Godwin-Austen, Janeway, and the proxy votes of Korczyn and Murray unanimously elected Antonio Culebras new President.

The new WNFo President, Antonio Culebras, presented a Strategic Plan Overview Draft in April 2004, at the WNFo Board Breakfast during the AAN meeting in San Francisco (32). The document represented a draft only, designed for the Board members of the WNFo. As one of the Board members, the WFN Secretary-Treasurer General, Richard Godwin-Austen replied on behalf of the WFN in a clear and well-structured letter dated 27 May 2004, and pointed out that the statements of mission as seen in the Strategic Plan had fundamentally changed the purpose of the WNFo, as stated in Article 1, in a way which he could not approve (33).

The relationship between the WFN and the WNFo became complicated during Culebras' presidency of the latter organization. As long as Toole was the WNFo President, much of the work focused upon establishing guidelines and bye-laws, obtaining a 501-C3 tax-exempt organization and initiating funding for the Endowed Lectures. In 2003, this part of the work was more or less completed, and we now had two independent organizations with an intimate internal connection, which had not yet been clarified. The WNFo agreed that the WNFo sole mission was to support the WFN (34).

As a tax-exempt organization in the USA, US laws bind the WNFo. In the special climate of the Patriot Act that was enacted after the September 11 attack, the laws had to be followed to the letter. This meant that the WNFo board had to be in full control of funds deposited in the WNFo account. Passing funds to the WFN treasury was therefore not an option.

The President of the WFN wrote to the WNFo President on 23 May 2004:

> The divergent views expressed about the function of WNFo rekindled the Trustees' anxiety about the relationship between the two organizations. I do not believe we can pretend the business as usual any longer without unequivocal clarification on the role

of WNFo as it relates to WFN. If the WNFo is, in fact, determined to pursue a course, which deviates from the original mission agreed upon at the time of inception, then it would be difficult for WFN to maintain a formal liaison. As you know, I have always been supportive of your effort as the new president of WNFo and am still hopeful that something more cohesive can be worked out between the two organizations. We must, however, have a clear understanding on what WNFo would do or would not do to the satisfaction of the WFN Fundraising Committee and Trustees if we were to sustain our amicable relationship. To this end, the current unhappy event may be a blessing in disguise if it helps initiate a constructive dialogue (34).

It did not. The financial climate for fund-raising projects of this kind has continued to deteriorate during the last ten years.

There has been a clear understanding that the WNFo is the fund-raising arm of the WFN in North America, and that the WNFo should not interfere with WFN fund-raising activities in the rest of the world. It has also become clear that the global fund-raising possibilities at present (2011) are dramatically different from how they were in 1999, when the WNFo was conceived.

In December 2005, Antonio Culebras decided to step down as WNFo President to devote his efforts to his newly elected position as president of the World Stroke Federation. At the WFN Strategy meeting in San Diego in April 2006, Michael Finkel was appointed new President of the WNFo.

References

1 **Poser CM.** The World Federation of Neurology: the formative period 1955–1961. Personal recollections. *J Neur Sci* 1993; **120**: 218–27.

2 **Bailey P.** WFN decentralization proposal. *J Neur Sci* 1965; **2**: 294–96.

3 **Van Bogaert L.** Meeting of the WFN Executive Committee. Closing remarks. *J Neur Sci* 1965; **2**: 296–97.

4 **Van Bogaert L.** Presidential Report. WFN Executive Committee Meeting. Vienna, 4 September 1965. *J Neur Sci* 1966; **3**: 444–50.

5 **Miller H.** Minutes of the Executive Committee of the World Federation of Neurology. Neurological Institute, New York 25 June 1967. *J Neurol Sci* 1968; **6**: 386–89.

6 **Miller H.** Minutes of the Meeting of the Executive Committee of the World Federation of Neurology. New York 21 September 1969. *J Neurol Sci* 1970; **10**: 504–05.

7 **Critchley M.** World Federation of Neurology. President's Report. *J Neurol Sci* 1970; **10**: 504–16.

8 **Olivarius B.** Minutes of the Meeting of the Council of Delegates. *J Neur Sci* 1976; **29**: 427–36.

9 **Walton J.** Minutes of the 1st Meeting of the Council of Delegates, Amsterdam 11 September 1977. *J Neur Sci* 1978; **36**: 289–300.

10 **Toole JF.** World Federation of Neurology: Meeting of Council of Delegates, Hamburg 10–11 June 1983. *J Neur Sci* 1984; **65**: 249–60.

11 **Toole JF.** Minutes of the Steering Committee 21 October 1989. *J Neur Sci* 1990; **97**: 325–36.

12 **Bruyn G.** Finance Committee Report. *J Neur Sci* 1990; **97**: 329.

13 Walton J. *The Spice of Life. From Northumbria to World Neurol. Chapter 20: The World Federation of Neurology.* Royal Society of Medicine Services, London 1993.

14 Rose FC. WFN News. *World Neurol* 1995; **10**(3/4): 1–3.

15 Rose FC. Recommendations for WFN Elections. *World Neurol* 1996; **11**(4): 5.

16 Chopra JS. Platform Programmes for Presidential Nominees. *World Neurol* 2000; **15**(4): 6.

17 Chopra JS. World Federation of Neurology Elections. Nominating Committee Recommendations. *World Neurol* 2004; **19**(4): 1.

18 Chopra JS. Platform Presentations of the Presidential Nominees. Platform Presentations of the First Vice-Presidential Nominees. *World Neurol* 2005; **20**(2): 7–10.

19 Spinney L. A Neurologist Strikes a Nerve. *Intelligent Life* 17 April 2010.

20 Hallett M. Candidates' Statements for President. *World Neurol* 2009; **24**(2): 1–7.

21 Toole JF. World Federation of Neurology: Information. Meeting of Council of Delegates, Hamburg 10–11 June 1983. *J Neurol Sci* 1984; **65**: 252.

22 Menken M. Neurological education. *World Neurol* 1990; **5**(1): 6–7.

23 Menken M. Neurological education. *World Neurol* 1991; **6**(4): 9.

24 Singhal B. Neurological Education in Asia and Oceania. *World Neurol* 1992; **7**(1): 14.

25 Rose FC. Resolution on neurological education. *World Neurol* 1995; **710**(11): 1–2.

26 Poeck, K. WFN to become active in continuing education. *World Neurol* 1996; **11**(1): 1.

27 Munsat T. WFN Initiatives. *World Neurol* 1998; **13**(3): 3.

28 Toole JF. Annual Report of the President for 1999. *World Neurol* 2000; **15**(1): 3–6.

29 Toole JF. Management Committee. *World Neurol* 1999; **14**(1): 6.

30 Toole JF. Introduction. Meeting invitation, 19 September 2000.

31 Toole JF. E-mail 4 October 2001 to Munsat and the WFN Trustees concerning Draft of letters for CME support.

32 Culebras A. World Neurology Foundation. Strategic Plan Overview—Draft. For WNF Board Breakfast 28 April 2004.

33 Godwin-Austen R. *World Neurol* Foundation—Strategic Plan. E-mail 27 May 2004.

34 Minutes from the Annual General Meeting/Council of Delegates 5 September 2004.

Chapter 4

The World Federation of Neurology Applied Research Committee

The World Federation of Neurology (WFN) Research Committee (re-named the WFN Applied Research Committee in 2010) is a cornerstone in the function of the Federation, and has been so since it was formed. It is based upon the Research Groups and their activities. Many sub-specialties in the clinical neurosciences started as WFN Research Groups, which later developed into international societies with their own congresses, journals, and administration. Some of them, like parkinsonism and related disorders, and headache and migraine, attract more participants to their congresses than do the WFN to the World Congresses. Other Research Groups are small, and the WFN Research Committee serves as an umbrella organization to link researchers in various parts of the world. For some neurologists, the link to the WFN Research Committee represents their strongest contact with international neurology. Together, the WFN Research Groups demonstrate the breadth and activities of contemporary clinical neurosciences.

The Research Groups are not a static part of the Federation. Since 1957, there have been more than 40 active Research Groups, but there were only 28 active Research Groups in 2011. Some have been disbanded, merged with others, or disappeared because of lack of interest. Several factors influence the viability of the groups. Contemporary development and new ideas in neurology are important, and the activity, or lack of activity, of the group leadership is essential. In 1960, when the WFN was new, there was apparently a need for a Research Group on Comparative Anatomy but there was no Research Group on Parkinsonism. Comparative anatomy is still an important field in the neurosciences, but few neurologists want it as a Research Group in clinical neurology any more. On the other hand, parkinsonism and related disorders have grown to become a major WFN Research Group.

The Problem Commissions

In 1957, an important mission for the new organization was to establish work groups or 'Problem Commissions' in the various sub-specialties and areas of interest in neurology to help develop international and interdisciplinary research projects. The Problem Commissions were supposed to organize separate specialized meetings and/or to take charge of specialized meetings within the framework of international congresses (1).

The Problem Commissions were formed during the first couple of years of the Federation's existence. Some of them were very active from the beginning, because of the importance of the topic. Some leaders such as Adolphe Franceschetti (neuro-ophthalmology) and David Klein (genetics) held international positions and had extensive networks in their fields and realized the future importance of the new global organization.

It was van Bogaert's idea that the Problem Commissions should represent the action programme of the WFN. 'Investigators in the same disciplines are getting to know one another, rub shoulders, and can communicate with one another directly or through our channels'. He also pointed out that it had now become possible for the WFN to contribute financially to these exchanges of men and ideas (2).

The role of the Problem Commissions in future World Congresses of Neurology

In his Presidential Report to the World Congress of Neurology in Vienna in 1965, Ludo van Bogaert was very clear in his vision of the role of the WFN Problem Commissions. His plan was that they should merge in a permanent organization, which should establish continuity and tradition in the organization of world congresses of neurology. 'It is the latter who actually have the ability to designate at a given moment the most qualified investigators in a particular field' (2).

However, there was no Research Committee during van Bogaert's Presidency. He realized that the Problem Commissions needed an overhead organization, and had named it the World Association of Neurological Commissions— WANC. The WANC was born in 1964, and van Bogaert saw it as a parallel organization to the WFN. John Walton also realized the importance of synchronization of the problem commissions, but saw it as an important element of the WFN (see Chapter 2, 'The WANC War').

By 1966, the WANC had been transformed into the Research Committee and a split in the Federation was avoided. The discussion of the position of the Research Groups had brought the WFN close to cleavage.

The WFN Research Committee 1966

The history of the Research Committee is different from that of the other WFN Committees. During the first WFN financial crisis, the Federation had considerable problems in establishing an adequate economy for the Problem Commissions. The Research Committee was established to provide a more stable WFN economy, but it also developed into an efficient medium to promote the scientific levels of various sub-specialties of neurology.

The Research Committee was founded by John Walton while he was Secretary of the Problem Commission on Neuromuscular Diseases. The first Chairman was Adolphe Franceschetti (1896–1968). He had already been formally elected Chairman of the concept of a WANC. David Klein (1908–1993), Franceschetti's colleague and close friend, had been elected Secretary-General of the WANC and became the Secretary-Treasurer of the new Committee. Both were close collaborators and based in Geneva. David Klein established a central bank account in Geneva. Franceschetti died suddenly in 1968 (Box 4.1).

Box 4.1 The obituary published in the *Journal of the Neurological Sciences*

Adolphe Franceschetti (1896–1968)

It was with profound regret that members of the World Federation of Neurology learned of the death of Professor Adolphe Franceschetti.

Born in Zurich in 1896, he became an international figure in the ophthalmological field, for he was a fluent linguist and a popular and enthusiastic participant in conferences and symposia. He had held the Chair of Ophthalmology at Geneva since 1933, and was Director of what must have been one of the most impressive eye-clinics in the world. Franceschetti, a dexterous operator, was among the pioneers in corneal grafting, and his colleagues today still make us of the trephine that he devised for this technique. It is perhaps in the field of genetically determined ophthalmological rarities where he is best known. The so-called mandibular-facial dysostosis is more familiar under the eponymous term Franceschetti's syndrome. The Institute of Medical Genetics of Switzerland originated as the result of his stimulus and endeavors, and he was the founder and editor of the *Journal de Génétique Humaine* in 1951. In 1954 he was President of the International Association for the Prevention of Blindness. For many years he has been a member of the International Council of Ophthalmology.

112 | THE HISTORY OF THE WORLD FEDERATION OF NEUROLOGY

> **Box 4.1 The obituary published in *Journal of the Neurological Sciences*** *(continued)*
>
> In the World Federation of Neurology he was the very active Secretary of the Research Group on Neuro-ophthalmology, and as such was responsible for the outstanding successful symposia held in Vienna (1964), Albi (1965) and in Montreal (1967). On the last-named occasion he was instrumental in arranging for the 3rd International Congress of Neuro-genetics and Neuro-ophthalmology to be held in Brussels in 1972. When the Research Committee of the WFN was constituted, Professor Franceschetti was appointed its first Chairman. He held this office up to the time of his death, and his colleagues had been looking forward to meeting him again at their May 1968 meeting in London.
>
> Professor Franceschetti was a man of forceful character, an eloquent and witty speaker, and an outstanding exponent of ophthalmology, particularly in its impingement upon the fields of genetics and neurology. His knowledge was both broad and deep, and ranged far outside of purely medical topics. His scholarship was displayed in his valuable library, so exceptional in magnitude and scope.
>
> The WFN owes much to Professor Franceschetti's dynamism, and he will be sadly missed in its councils.
>
> Macdonald Critchley
>
> President, World Federation of Neurology
>
> The obituary published in *Journal of the Neurological Sciences* volume 6: Adolphe Franceschetti (1896–1968), pp. 599–600. Copyright Elsevier (1968).

At the World Congress of Neurology in New York in 1969, Ernst Frauchiger (1903–1975), who was the Director of the Institute of Animal Neurology in Berne, Switzerland, was appointed his successor.

The Transformation of the Problem Commissions into Research Groups

The Research Committee (formerly World Association of Neurological Commissions) had its first meeting in Geneva, 1–2 July 1966. After considerable discussion, it was agreed that the World Association of Neurological Commissions should not continue in its present form, but be replaced by a Standing Research Committee of the WFN, to be made up mainly of the secretaries of the WFN Problem Commissions, now renamed Research Groups. The Executive Committee (renamed the Council of Delegates) of the WFN approved this. The Research Committee was entitled to elect its own Chairman and Secretary-Treasurer.

One reason for the reorganization was the financial constraints of the WFN. The compromise involved that each Problem Commission, now a Research Group, should charge a subscription not only to its founding members, but also to the associate members who would be recruited by each group on a worldwide basis. There was a hope that the income should cover the expenses of the Research Committee. However, fewer than half of the members of the individual research groups ever paid their subscriptions and the income was inadequate even to cover the secretarial expenses of Franceschetti and Klein. The financial problems of the WFN therefore remained. At the meeting of the Research Committee in New York in 1969, it was clear that insufficient funds had been obtained, and it had not been possible to give financial support to any of the Research Groups. Still, the worst part of the crisis was apparently over.

The Research Groups and the WFN economy

David Klein proposed in 1969 that the subscription for individual members of Research Groups should be raised to $5 annually. After some discussion, it was agreed that the present subscription of $2 should stand (in addition to the annual dues to the WFN). It was also accepted that individual Research Groups would be at liberty to apply to grant-giving organizations, and particularly to help them to organize meetings and symposia.

Klein administered the budget of the WFN Research Committee from Geneva in a very effective way. The secretariat was subsidized only by the dues from individual members of the groups. The funds were, however, too small to allow any major initiatives to be undertaken, and travel expenses of members to meetings were not covered. The WFN was therefore unable to support the Research Groups financially, which was a source of continuing disappointment (3).

During the World Congress in Amsterdam in 1977, George Bruyn proposed to discontinue the central collection of individual subscriptions. Instead, the Research Groups should attempt to raise sufficient funds for the support of their activities, and 10% of this should be paid to WFN central funds to support the administrative costs of the Research Committee (4).

John Walton and Armand Lowenthal made another attempt to encourage the Research Groups to raise sufficient funds. It was decided that a major objective of the WFN Research Groups should be, whenever possible and appropriate, to promote the establishment of new international societies for specialties within the neurosciences. These new societies were later invited to become corporate members of the Research Committee with the payment of an annual subscription. They could then be represented in the Research Committee with one vote. This led to the inclusion of organizations like the International Stroke Society, the Research Group on Multiple Sclerosis, and other similar bodies. The members of the Research Committee are therefore either representatives of a Research Group, or represent an affiliated organization.

The WFN policy concerning Research Groups was that travel grants might be given to chairmen of the groups, but the Research Groups should be self-supporting financially and raise funds to support their own activities.

It was decided in 1982 that subscription of founding and associate membership of the Research Groups should remain at 20 Swiss francs. In Hamburg 1985, the Council of Delegates and the Research Committee eliminated the individual subscription of members of the Research Groups to replace them with a standard assessment or an overhead charge on grants solicited by the Research Groups.

In 1987, the Third World Medical Research Foundation announced two grants to further the work of the WFN. The Third World Medical Research Foundation sponsors scientific studies and education of neglected nutritional, toxic, and other diseases that affect large numbers of people in underdeveloped parts of the world. Emphasis is directed toward research on disorders of the brain and nervous system, and research is supported (5). The first grant of US$500 was to underwrite the secretarial, administrative, and postal expenses of the Research Group on Neuromuscular Diseases, while the other grant, also US$500, was to underwrite the comparable costs of the Research Committee of the WFN.

The Research Committee (from 2010 the Applied Research Committee)

The Research Committee has become increasingly important both in coordinating the interplay between the Federation and the individual Research Groups, and for its position in the formation of scientific programmes for the world congresses. The Research Committee is a standing committee of the WFN. The President with the advice and approval of the Trustees appoints its Chair. Members of this Committee consist of the chairpersons of the various Research Groups. It is a fundamental and most important part of WFN activities. The strength of the WFN lies to a great degree in the breadth of its neurological spread.

When John Walton took over as Chairman of the Research Committee in 1977, he reviewed the position of the Committee and organized its written responsibilities (6,7). The Research Committee itself has changed from a quasi-autonomous entity with its own statutes to an integral WFN committee subject to the new WFN constitution just like any other committee. It plays a vital role in helping to formulate, for instance, the scientific programme of each World Congress of Neurology.

The transformation of the WFN Research Committee

As described earlier, the structure of the WFN was modified when the WFN developed corporate status. While the Research Committee was relatively independent, it now developed into an integral WFN committee subject to the new WFN constitution just like any other Standing Committee. Its main function and the relationship to the Research Groups remained as before.

When Roger Rosenberg took over as Chair of the WFN Research Committee in 2001, he put forward an important initiative, the formation of a Research Committee website 'Research Advances in Neurology', with the intent of developing an electronic syllabus emphasizing 'New and Emerging Neuro-Therapeutics: Results of Basic and Clinical Research'. This initiative was approved unanimously, and it also served as a basis for the scientific programme at the World Congress of Neurology in Bangkok 2009.

Chairs of the WFN Research Committee

Adolphe Franceschetti (Geneva, Switzerland) 1966–1968

Ernst Frauchiger (Bern, Switzerland) 1969–1975

David Klein (Geneva, Switzerland) as Secretary-Treasurer General until 1985. Frauchiger died in 1975.

R. Fankhauser (Bern) was acting Chairman until the new Chairman was elected in 1977.

Armand Lowenthal became both Secretary and Treasurer, and David Klein an honorary life member of the Research Committee.

John Walton (Newcastle, UK) 1977–1989. He was appointed Chairman of the Research Committee at the World Congress in Amsterdam 1977, with Armand Lowenthal as Secretary. The office of the Treasurer of the Research Committee was disbanded in 1985.

Klaus Poeck (Aachen, Germany) 1989–1997

Theodore Munsat (Boston, USA) 1997–2001

Roger Rosenberg (Dallas, USA) 2001–2009

Donna S. Bergen (Chicago, USA) and Philip Gorelick (Chicago, USA) (advisor) 2010–

Structural problems of commission organization

The Problem Commissions had only minor economic problems during the first few years of the Federation. Financial constraints appeared around 1965, and represented a special problem because the groups were based upon international collaboration. International travelling is time-consuming, expensive, and complicated, and the long distances made it difficult to create international collaborative groups. The new research centres in Japan, Australia, South America, and India offered additional communication problems. Many of the WFN Problem Commissions were therefore twins, with one Eastern and one Western half. Usually, the Eastern included Europe and the Asian-Oceanian Region, and the Western the Americas.

The major Problem Commissions had a President and a Secretary-General, sometimes with special secretaries for the eastern and for the western hemisphere, respectively.

The first Problem Commissions

After the initial period, the economy of the WFN became insecure. The meetings of the Problem Commissions were often held with support and hospitality from universities, research foundations, and drug companies and to a great extent also personal expenditure to meet the costs of travel and accommodation.

The spectrum of neurological problems reflected in the list of Commissions is based upon clinical aspects and less upon basic neurosciences. Parkinsonism was apparently not regarded as a research problem when the first Problem Commissions in neurology were set up. In 1957, Arvid Carlsson, who shared the Nobel Prize in physiology and medicine in 2000, demonstrated that L-dopa and its main metabolite dopamine could reverse the Parkinson-like akinesia that developed in reserpinized animals. Possible therapeutic consequences in neurology were not realized until Cotzias' demonstration of transient benefit of Parkinsonism after injection of L-dopa in 1967 (8). Melvin Yahr founded the WFN Research Group on Extrapyramidal Disorders in 1973.

Colleagues initiated the first Problem Commissions with an insight into the new organization; they had international networks and their research interest was the analysis of clinical aspects. Basic research in neurosciences had to wait. Geographical neurology, aphasia, and neurochemistry were among the first.

Problem Commission on Geographical Neurology, Statistics and Epidemiology

The first WFN Problem Commission with clinicians and neuroscientists with one focused interest was 'Geographical Neurology, Statistics and Epidemiology'. It was established in Rome on 8 June 1959. It reflected the importance of neuroepidemiological research, initially specially related to multiple sclerosis. Leonard Kurland, then Chief of the Neuroepidemiology Branch of the National Institute of Neurological Diseases and Blindness (NINDB), John Kurtzke, and Kay Hyllested of Copenhagen primarily organized it, for the purpose of sponsoring a geomedical conference on multiple sclerosis, which was held in Copenhagen in June 1959. Kurland reviewed the past activities of the commission at the congress in Rome in 1961. The Commission had a third conference on geographic neurology in Copenhagen in 1963, also with the main emphasis on multiple sclerosis, but with a broader view on geographic neurology with the focus on several chronic neurological disorders like parkinsonism, kuru, and amyotrophic lateral sclerosis (9,10).

A global organization on Geographical Neurology, as was the Commission's original name, necessitated extensive networking, sponsored by the WFN. Thus, Professor Ernest Donald Acheson (1926–2010) (Southampton, UK), an outstanding epidemiologist, visited Australia, New Zealand, and South Africa. In his report to the President of the WFN, he reviewed comparative studies of multiple sclerosis and other demyelinating diseases in these countries.

The activity of this commission was primarily focused upon the geography of multiple sclerosis, but Kurland also pointed out the need for similar survey procedures on cerebrovascular disease and parkinsonism.

The Problem Commission on Geographical Neurology was later disbanded and integrated in the Research Group on Neuroepidemiology. This Research Group publishes the journal *Neuroepidemiology*. It became clear that multiple sclerosis needed a special Research Group (see 'Multiple Sclerosis Research Group', p. 131).

Problem Commission of Neurochemistry

The second Problem Commission was the Commission of Neurochemistry. It was organized by Armand Lowenthal, Georges Edgar, and Charles Poser and had its first meeting in Antwerp in September 1959 (Fig. 4.1). Among the founding fathers were Wallace Tourtellotte (USA), Judah Quastel (USA), John L. Cummings (UK), Armand Lowenthal (Belgium), E. Pearse, Derek Richter (UK), Lars Svennerholm (Sweden), Jordi Folch-Pi (USA/Spain), Saul Korey (USA), G. Brante (Sweden), Ludo van Bogaert (WFN), H. Bauer (Germany), Georges Edgar (Belgium), and Charles Poser (WFN) (1).

When Armand Lowenthal initiated this work, neurochemistry appeared more homogeneous than anticipated, but it turned out that several neurochemists were more engaged in basic neurochemistry than they were in clinical neurochemistry. The Problem Commission of Neurochemistry organized a Symposium in Gothenburg in 1962 and decided to allow 'an extensive number of neurochemists to join'. The members of the commission then met in Antwerp

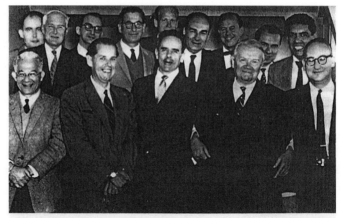

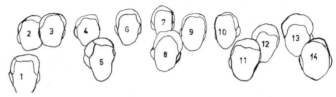

Fig. 4.1 First meeting of the Commission of Neurochemistry, Antwerp September 29/30 1959.

1. F. Quastel (US), 2. W. Tourtellotte (US), 3. J. Cummings (UK), 4. A. Lowenthal (Belgium), 5. E. Pearse (UK), 6. D. Richter (UK), 7. L. Svennerholm (Sweden), 8. J. Folch-Pi (US), 9. S. Korey (US), 10. G Brante (Sweden), 11. L. van Bogaert (WFN), 12. H. Bauer (Germany), 13. G. Edgar (The Netherlands), 14. C. Poser.

Reprinted from *J Neurol Sci*, 120, W. Tourtellotte and C. Poser, The World Federation of Neurology: the formative period. Personal Recollections 1955–1961, 218. Copyright (1993), with permission from Elsevier.

in 1963 and agreed to continue its activity and perhaps acquire a more permanent and lasting status.

There was an attempt in 1962 to organize an international society of neurochemistry without the Problem Commission of Neurochemistry being officially recognized. An appeal was launched to all neurochemists to create a truly international organization. A major question proved to be if the neurochemists interested in clinical neurology could obtain equal rights with the pure neurochemists (11).

There were many threads, which contributed to the creation of the International Society of Neurochemistry. In addition to the activities of the

Mental Health Research Fund and the WFN, the first International Congress of Biochemistry was held in 1949 in London and included neurochemical contributions. Discussions amongst Japanese scientists at a meeting in 1958 led to the formation of the first Neurochemical society, the Japanese Society for Neurochemistry, in 1962. It was decided in 1981 that the International Societies (International, American, European) for Neurochemistry would participate in the activities of the Research Group and have appointed representatives, but the WFN Research Group on Neurochemistry was disbanded.

Problem Commission on the History of Neurology

The Problem Commission on the History of Neurology is also among the oldest, and has continuously had high scientific activity. C.D. O'Malley first chaired it. The purpose of the Commission was the creation of documentation and study centres, the establishment of an inventory of materials for the history of neurology, preparation of historical exhibits for exhibition at neurological congresses, organization of symposia on the history of neurology, and creation of fellowships. The first symposium was held in Varenna, Italy, in 1961, the next in Münster in 1962. Over the years, the Commission (Research Group) has organized several successful historical meetings, many of them related to the World Congresses of Neurology. The present Chairman is George York (Fiddletown, CA, USA). This Research Group is an Applied Research Group, and has its own journal.

Problem Commission of Language Disorders (Aphasia/ Cognitive Disorders Research Group)

The Problem Commission of Language Disorders was one of the first Problem Commissions. Several colleagues objected to the name, and it was then renamed 'Problem Commission of Aphasiology'. Georg Schaltenbrand claimed that it was founded in Heidelberg, and Macdonald Critchley admitted that it was founded 'somewhere in the Black Forest'. This commission had its first meeting at Villa Monastero, Varenna, at Lake Como, 5–7 May 1966. The Chair was Eberhard Bay from Düsseldorf, who became the Secretary of the Problem Commission on Language Disorders, later Aphasiology. Macdonald Critchley gave the opening speech on 'Nomenclature and definitions in aphasiology'. Bay then talked about 'Classification of the aphasias', and the third speaker was Arthur Benton (Iowa), who talked about 'The examination of the aphasic patient'.

The proceedings from the meeting in Varenna were published, as were proceedings from the Princeton meeting in 1965 on 'Brain mechanisms underlying speech and language'. The second edition of Lord Brain's *Aphasia, Apraxia and Agnosia* was published by Butterworth in 1965, as were other books on this topic.

In 1967, Germaine Ribière feared an overlap might occur between the Research Group on Developmental Neurology, and the new Research Group on Developmental Dyslexia and Word Illiteracy. That group had been founded in 1968 and had its first meeting at the Texas Scottish Rite Hospital, Dallas, during Macdonald Critchley's presidency. The group focused upon *specific developmental dyslexia,* and formulated adequate definitions of dyslexia. John Walton suggested that the two groups should collaborate in joint activities. The Research Group on Dyslexia was disbanded in 1979, and members of the group were invited to join the Research Group on Aphasiology.

This group developed smoothly into the WFN Research Group on Aphasia/ Cognitive Disorders. Thomas H. Bak (Centre for Clinical Brain Sciences, Edinburgh, Scotland) is the present Chair, and Facundo Manes, Institute of Cognitive Neurology (Buenos Aires, Argentina) Co-Chair. The main objectives of this Research Group are:

1 to unite the leading researchers of the field, providing a forum for cutting edge scientific debates and exchange of ideas, in particular at our biennial meetings;

2 to raise the profile and presence of aphasiology and cognitive and behavioural neurology at neurological meetings and in neurological literature;

3 to foment interest in the disorders of language, cognition, and behaviour among young neurologists worldwide and to nurture young talent in the field;

4 to establish and maintain close links with the WFN and its research groups as well as with other relevant organizations (e.g. European Federation of Neurological Societies, EFNS);

5 to provide expert guidance to clinicians, from informal advice to clinical guidelines and recommendations.

This Research Group organized a well-attended Biennial Meeting in 2010 at the island of Heybeliada in the Sea of Marmara, near Istanbul. Marsel Mesulam (USA) gave the opening lecture on 'The Language Network in Primary Progressive Aphasia'. Important issues were the comparison between vascular and neurodegenerative aphasias, and how to establish cognitive neurology clinics in countries with different populations, disease profiles, cultures, and languages. The Research Group also initiated the Forum of Young Researchers in 2009 to promote interest in cognitive neurology among young scientists and clinicians. It had its first gathering at the Istanbul meeting.

THE WORLD FEDERATION OF NEUROLOGY APPLIED RESEARCH COMMITTEE | **121**

Research Group on Neuromuscular Diseases

In 1964, John Walton proposed to the WFN President, Ludo van Bogaert, that the WFN should establish a Problem Commission on Neuromuscular Diseases. The commission was formally set up in Newcastle in January 1965. John Walton was elected chairman and secretary. Irena Hausmanowa-Petrusewicz of Warsaw, Christian Coërs of Brussels, Raymond Garcin of Paris, and Werner Trojaborg of Copenhagen, representing Fritz Buchtal, were present at the meeting.

The Problem Commission (later Research Group) of Neuromuscular Diseases soon developed into one of the major Research Groups of the WFN (12). It expanded the original classification of disorders of the muscle and organized a series of successful quadrennial international congresses on muscle diseases. Reports on histochemical fibre type nomenclature of human skeletal muscle, on the terminology and techniques with respect to tissue culture studies, and on spinal muscular atrophies were published in the 1970s. The First International Congress on Neuromuscular Diseases took place in Milan in 1971, the Second in Newcastle upon Tyne in 1974. Starting from 1978, these congresses became quadrennial: Montreal 1978, Marseilles 1982, Los Angeles 1986, Munich 1990, Kyoto 1994, Adelaide 1998, Vancouver 2002, Istanbul 2006, and Naples 2010. During this period, the development in our understanding of the basis of muscle diseases increased dramatically, and many investigators felt that a four-year interval between meetings was too long. In 1995, a new multidisciplinary society, the World Muscle Society (WMS), was formed. Since 1996, the WMS has organized annual muscle congresses and has its own journal, *Neuromuscular Disorders*, which is the official journal of the WMS. The first annual WMS congress took place in London in 1996. The WFN Research Group on neuromuscular disorders selected Naples for the International Congress on Neuromuscular Diseases in 2010, and it was organized under the auspices of the WFN. Professor Gerard Said (Paris) was the chair of this Research Group.

Research Group on Comparative Neuroanatomy

This is one of the oldest WFN Research Groups. It had two sections. Professor Heinz Stephan (Frankfurt, Germany) chaired the eastern, and Professor Howard A. Matzke (Kansas City, USA) the western. Heinz Stephan organized several symposia relevant to clinical neurology. When they met in 1965, there were 14 members and 75 corresponding members. The commission was actively involved in research on the methodology of the morphological differentiation of the normal human thalamus and on comparative anatomy, and on the nomenclature of the central nervous system valid for all mammals (13). This Problem Commission was later disbanded.

Research Group on Neuro-anaesthesiology

Gilbert Glaser (Montreal) was the first President, and there were an eastern and a western section. In the absence of major financial support, Glaser and Terry recommended decentralization, with two self-supporting sections. The commission was active from the beginning. It organized successful symposia, but it was soon clear that neuro-anaesthesiology was much more closely related to neurological surgery than to neurology. It has now disbanded as a WFN Research Group.

Problem Commission on Developmental Neurology

Stéphane Thieffry and Germaine Ribière (Paris) chaired this problem commission, which changed its status and function over the years. Its first name was 'infantile neurology', which was then changed to 'developmental neurology'; it was considered to be a basic science, especially in problems of language development. In 1967, Germaine Ribière feared an overlap might occur with the new Research Group on Developmental Dyslexia and Word Illiteracy, which was later disbanded.

The WFN Problem Commission on Developmental Neurology was renamed the Research Group for Neuropaediatrics, which was proposed in 1968 and had its first business meeting in Vienna in 1971 and also met at Marianske Lasni, Czechoslovakia. The first official session was in Prague and Marienbad in 1972, mainly thanks to the work of the Secretary, Professor I. Lesny of Prague. The first session dealt with the classification of cerebral palsy.

In consultation with the International Society for Pediatric Neurology, it was agreed that the International Society for Pediatric Neurology will be represented on the Research Committee by its Secretary-General. The Research Group on Paediatric Neurology continued to be active, largely in Eastern Europe, while there is today no WFN Research Group on Neuropaediatrics. The International Society for Pediatric Neurology (the International Child Neurology Association) is represented on a corporate basis in the WFN Research Committee as a group affiliated to the committee.

Research Group on Neuro-oncology

This Problem Commission, with Klaus Zülch as Chairman, worked mainly to establish contacts among the members, and organized a separate symposium at the World Congress of Neurology in Vienna in 1965. It has now disbanded. It was decided in 1965 that the *Acta Neuropathologica* should be not only a journal of the Problem Commission of Neuropathology, but also of the WFN Problem Commission of Neuro-Oncology.

Research Group of Neurogenetics

Professor David Klein, Geneva (1908–1985), was founding chairman and secretary of this Problem Commission, which had its own official journal, *Journal de Génétique Humaine*. It had from the beginning a close collaboration with the Problem Commission on Neuro-ophthalmology. For a long time, Klein and Franceschetti worked together at Franceschetti's department of ophthalmology in Geneva, and they shared an interest in genetics and neuro-ophthalmology. In 1959, Klein was appointed Professor Extraordinaire, and in 1970 he became full Professor of Medical Genetics. Both were active in developing the WFN Research Committee and had a unique collaboration.

In 1988, Anita Harding was looking for WFN research activities in neurogenetics. John Walton recommended that the Research Group should be reorganized within the neurogenetics field, and that Eva Andermann (Montreal Neurological Hospital & Institute, Canada) should become the new chair, which she still is (2011).

The Research Group does not do research per se, but serves as a forum for meetings and exchange of research-related information. Part of its programme has been symposia organized in conjunction with the annual meeting of the American Academy of Neurology.

Problem Commission on Neuro-ophthalmology and Neuro-otology

Adolphe Franceschetti, Geneva, (1896–1968) became the Chairman of Ophthalmology in 1933, and remained in that position until his death in 1968. He was the founder and editor of the journal in 1951, to be followed by David Klein. Franceschetti organized a series of successful symposia on neurogenetics and neuro-ophthalmology (Vienna 1964, Albi 1965, and Montreal 1967).

Like several WFN Research Groups, the Research Group on neuro-ophthalmology had two sections, the eastern, which was mainly European, and the western, including the Americas and the Asian-Oceania region. Franceschetti was the secretary of the eastern section of the commission, while Frank W. Newell was responsible for the western section (14). The associate and corresponding members of the Problem Commission of the western section decided in 1962 to meet at the Pan-American Ophthalmological Association or the Pan-Pacific Asian Academy meetings, while those of the eastern could convene at meetings of the European Society of Ophthalmology. One consequence was that many ophthalmologists with an interest in neuro-ophthalmology found ophthalmology meetings more attractive for their purpose.

The WFN Research Group on Neuro-ophthalmology

It has since developed into the Research Group on Neuro-ophthalmology and Neuro-otology. G Michael Halmagyi (Royal Prince Alfred Hospital, Camperdown, Australia) is the present Chair, but there has not been any contact with WFN within the last two years.

Research Group on Neuropathology

In 1959, a handful of neuropathologists came together at the Hospice de la Salpetrière to discuss the future training in neuropathology. Franz Seitelberger was elected Chairman of the commission. In 1961, *Acta Neuropathologica* was founded as the organ of the WFN Problem Commission of Neuropathology, Comparative Neuropathology, and Neuro-oncology. *Acta Neuropathologica* became the official journal, and Seitelberger the Editor-in-Chief for a period also participated in the editing for the Problem Commission of Comparative Neuropathology. The WFN contributed towards the expenses of publishing.

The Research Group on Neuropathology has been active since the beginnings of the WFN. It has participated actively in the international congresses of the WFN as well as in other national meetings or international symposia. At the World Congress in Sydney (2005), it organized a workshop with the aim of updating neuropathological topics such as neurodegenerative diseases, muscle, or brain tumour pathology. This workshop was completed with collaborative and integrated activity presenting cases and hot problems in clinical neuropathology.

Historically, the European Congresses in Neuropathology started in Vienna (Austria) followed by Warsaw (Poland), Verona (Italy), Berlin (Germany), Paris (France), Barcelona (Spain), Helsinski (Finland), and Amsterdam (Holland). The group organized several international symposia in neuropathology. The WFN sponsored its official organ, *Acta Neuropathologica*. An International Society of Neuropathology was established and became affiliated to the WFN as Corporate Members, but the Research Group on Neuropathology remained in the WFN. The most recent (2011) chair was Dr Felix Cruz-Sanchez, Barcelona. Unfortunately, he died the same year and the WFN has not yet been informed about his successor. The Research Group on Comparative Neuropathology had previously engulfed the Research Group on Comparative Neuroanatomy. Professor R. Fankhauser, Bern, was the first chairman and secretary of that group, which had close contact with veterinary neuropathology. It does not exist as a separate Research Group.

Research Group on Neuroradiology

No one could predict the dramatic development in neuroradiology when this Problem Commission was formed in 1960. The first Chairman was Professor Herman Fischgold (Paris), with Lucien Appel (Antwerp) as Assistant Secretary. Professor Fischgold organized Journées de Neuroradiologie in Paris in 1962, supported by the WFN. The Journées were very successful, with 250 participants.

The Commission decided to devote its efforts to the following projects and resolutions:

1 establishment of criteria for training in neuroradiology;

2 establishment of a unified nomenclature of descriptive neuroradiology;

3 establishment of a unified index of neurologic publications;

4 adoption of a unified nomenclature in the use of radioisotopes in neurology and neurosurgery. The name of *gamma-encephalography* to be applied to this technique was recommended by the Commission;

5 establishment of a registry of complications of neuroradiological procedures;

6 investigation of the possibility of applying the newer techniques of high-energy therapy to neurological problems;

7 establishment of a programme of mutual collaboration with the organizational committee of the Sixth Symposium Neuroradiologicum.

The last (2011) chair was Jean Tamraz, Beirut, Lebanon. Unfortunately, the WFN has had no contact with this Research Group for the last two years.

Neuroimaging Research Group

At the World Congress of Neurology in Kyoto in 1981, Franz Gerstenbrand proposed formation of a Research Group on Computerized Tomography and Neuroimaging. The Research Committee agreed on its formation. It was later renamed the Research Group on Neuroimaging.

Joseph C. Masdeu invited neurologists currently involved in functional neuroimaging, and particularly in functional MRI and PET, to participate more actively in the Research Group. The group has been increasingly concerned about neuroimaging training, and the role of neurologists in endovascular procedures.

Joseph C. Masdeu (Bethesda, USA) is the present chair (2011). They organized a Neuroimaging Symposium for the 2009 World Congress in Bangkok. The relevant page of the WFN website, written and maintained by the Neuroimaging Research Group, is one of the most visited on the WFN website.

Problem Commission on Tropical Neurology

This was one of the first groups to be organized. Van Bogaert had pointed out that it merited WFN support more than any other sector of neurological sciences. It had two sections, one for the west (chairmen Walter E. Maffei and W.L. Sanvito) and one for the east (chairman Hatai Chitanwudth).

The clinical problems in tropical neurology made it necessary to establish a bigger framework, with one centre in Asia (Thailand), one in South America, and one in Africa. The centre in Thailand, supported by the NINDB, was active in investigations on parasitic diseases of the nervous system. The South American group focused on tropical neuropathology, neurocysticercosis, and Chagas' disease. The African centre worked on trypanosomiasis and nutritional neuropathies and collaborated with the WHO centres in Sierra Leone, Ghana, Cameroon, and Liberia. Professor B.O. Osuntokun (Ibadan, Nigeria) became the leader of the African research activities in tropical neurology.

In 1961, the WFN organized in Buenos Aires an international symposium on Tropical Neurology. At the 7th International Congress of Tropical Medicine in Rio de Janeiro in 1963, the WFN Problem Commission on Tropical Neurology had a separate symposium on typical forms of the encephalitides. The western division of the Problem Commission established sub-commissions in Sao Paulo, Rio de Janeiro, Buenos Aires, Montevideo, and Lima. It gradually became clear that tropical neurology was such a large field of neurology that the meetings developed into International Congresses of Tropical Neurology.

In his lifetime, Professor Osuntokun (Ibadan, Nigeria) was an active organizer of activities, also with close contacts to the WHO.

The Chair in 2011 was Oscar Del Brutto (Guayaquil, Ecuador). Unfortunately, the WFN has had no contact with this Research Group for the last two years.

In 1961, India took back Goa, which had been a Portuguese colony. Noshir Wadia, who had participated in the Congress of Tropical Neurology in South America, was arrested in Lisbon on his way home, and was in a Portuguese prison in Lisbon for 2 weeks (see Chapter 8).

Research Group on Ataxia

This Research Group succeeded the Research Group on Heredoataxia, of which David Klein (1908–1985) was one of the founding fathers. Andre Barbeau, who was the Chair, died in 1986. Before his death, he had suggested that this Research Group should become a Research Group on Ataxia with Robert D. Currier (Jackson, Ms, USA) and Anita Harding (London, UK) as co-secretaries.

The group organized a satellite symposium on inherited ataxias in 1999. It was focused on the molecular pathogenesis of Friedreich's ataxia and the role of frataxin. The current status of transgenic models and current efforts at therapy were discussed.

The present Chair (2011) is Alexandra Durr, Hôpital de la Salpêtrière, (Paris, France).

Research Group on Autonomic Disorders

The present Chair (2011) is Roy Freeman, Harvard Medical School (Boston, USA).

Research Group on Clinical Neuropharmacology

The Council of Delegates in Buenos Aires in 1997 approved this Research Group. The present Chair is Amos Korczyn, Tel Aviv University Medical School, Israel.

Research Group on Dementia

The research group on dementia was started in 1983 under the direction of Dr B. Tomlinson, M. Roth, and Dr G. Blessed. These pioneer neurologists in the dementias from the Newcastle Group extended this initiative to include American colleagues and specifically Dr Robert Katzman. The group therefore formed with primarily two geographic foci, one based in the USA and one in Europe, with the scope however to reach the rest of the world in regard to stimulating research and epidemiological work into dementias. The first conference was held in Hamburg, Germany, in the same year and the results of this free-standing meeting resulted in a publication about the direction of the local organizers and editor, Dr Poeck.

Over the following years, the group has organized several satellite meetings to coincide with the World Congress of Neurology. Since the first meeting held in conjunction with the 13th World Congress of Neurology in Hamburg, the meetings have been held in different European cities such as Helsinki and Vancouver under the direction of Professor Luigi Amaducci from Florence and Katherine Bick from the NIH. Activities of the group have extended to Africa and South America with meetings in Buenos Aires, Johannesburg, Nairobi, and Marrakesh.

The group reached out to World Societies of Neurology and Neurosciences, organizing conferences to coincide with meetings of Alzheimer Disease International (ADI) as well as the Society of Neuroscientists of Africa (SONA). The first such meeting with the SONA organization was held in Marrakesh in 1995.

Since then under the leadership of Peter Whitehouse, the group has extended its activities in attempting to harmonize the approval process of anti-dementia drugs worldwide in order to speed up this process. More recently the group has established an educational fellowship in the name of Professor Luigi Amaducci, one of the first chairs of the group, with the purpose to stimulate research in dementias in promising young investigators. Recipients so far have been young investigators from Venezuela and Columbia.

At present, the group is maintaining its worldwide scope under the leadership of Dr Raul Arizaga in Buenos Aires, where local regional meetings have been held under the sponsorship of the Research Group on Dementia. These activities are continuing to extend, and a meeting on cognitive function was planned for October 2013 in conjunction with the Vascular Dementia Congress in Athens, Greece. The WFN-RGD co-organized the Symposium 'Brain Ageing and Dementia in Developing Countries' held in Nairobi, Kenya, on 5–7 December 2012.

World Federation of Neurology Research Group on Dementia (WFN-RGD) 2011 report

I Organizational track

- To December 2011 the WFN-RGD had 280 members.
- During 2012 the authorities' renewal will take place by a vote of the Executive Committee.

II Scientific—academic track

- On May 2011 the 3rd WFN-RGD Latin American Meeting at the National Academy of Medicine was held in Buenos Aires with more than 400 registered attendees (neurologists, psychiatrists, geriatricians and neuropsychologists.
- The WFN-RGD is co-organizing the Symposium 'Brain Ageing and Dementia in Developing Countries' to be held in December in Nairobi, Kenya on 5–7 December 2012.
- The WFN-RGD is co-organizing the First European Cognitive Impairment Meeting in Athens on 17–20 October 2013.

III Educational track

As part of the frame agreement signed with the Argentine National Institute for Social Services for Retired and Pensioners, a long distance course about 'Cognition and Behavior: anatomical and neurochemical basis' directed at general practitioners, neurologists, psychiatrists, and geriatricians was organized. More than 900 professionals were registered and more than 600 of them took and approved a multiple-choice examination.

THE WORLD FEDERATION OF NEUROLOGY APPLIED RESEARCH COMMITTEE | **129**

IV Communicational track

The WFN-RGD web page was renewed and actualized with announcements, news, meetings, and congress agendas with the aim of improving the external presence and the internal communication of the WFN-RGD. In 2012 www.wfn-rgd.org will be linked to the WFN webpage.

Conexión (Connection), a printed newsletter in Spanish is distributed to 10 000 neurologists, psychiatrists, and geriatricians. Two issues were distributed during 2011. Four issues are planned for 2012.

An agreement signed with the *Journal of Alzheimer's Disease* allowed WFN-RGD members free access to the electronic edition for one year. Renewal of the agreement is planned to be signed.

V Socio-sanitary and health policies track

A renewal of the frame agreement was signed with the Argentine National Institute for Social Services for Retired and Pensioners, which deals with the social and health services for more than 4 million individuals older than 65 years.

Research Group on Environmental Neurology (formerly Neurotoxicology)

There was previously a Research Group on Industrial and Environmental Neurology. It was relatively active, and organized symposia on industrial and environmental neurology, mainly in Czechoslovakia. Eliska Klimkova-Deutschova, who was the Secretary, died in 1981. Professor Edgar Lukas who very successfully organized the 4th International Congress on Industrial and Environmental Neurology in Prague 1984 reconstituted the group.

Research Group on Neurotoxicology

The name was later changed to the WFN Research Group on Environmental Neurology. This was a multidisciplinary research group composed of neurologists and neuropathologists. It was initiated and organized by Professor Leon Roizin (USA) and approved by the WFN in 1977. Its membership was later expanded in order to include research scientists from other multidisciplinary bio-medical sciences related to neurotoxicology. During his WFN Presidency, Richard Masland held preliminary discussions with Drs Lukas and Roizin in New York. As a result of the discussions, it was recommended to merge the two Research groups, the WFN Neurotoxicology and the Occupational Neurology Research Groups, which was approved in Hamburg 1985. The present Chairman is Leon Prockop, University of South Florida, Tampa, USA.

The goals of this Research Group are to promote clinical research and education in all matters to do with the adverse effects of environmental substances/events, including neurotoxins, upon the nervous system. These include, but are not limited to, heavy metals, volatile hydrocarbons, and insecticides and pesticides. Humans may be exposed to these substances/events in industrial/occupations situations or as a result of terrorism.

Research Group on Huntington's Disease

The present Chairman (2011) is Raymund Roos (Leiden, the Netherlands). The Research Group on Huntington's disease was assisted financially by generous contributions from the Committee to Combat Huntington's Disease, leading to important research projects. There were successful World Congresses of Huntington's disease in Dresden, Germany, in 2007 and in Vancouver, Canada, in 2009.

These congresses are the major congresses on Huntington's disease with presentations from scientists, neurologists, and other clinicians as well as the wider Huntington's disease community, including family members and support groups. They are a combined initiative of the WFN Research Group on Huntington's Disease, the International HD Association, and the Huntington Society of Canada.

Intensive Care Neurology Research Group

Daniel Hanley, Johns Hopkins Hospital, Baltimore, is the current chair of the Intensive Care Research Group.

Migraine and Headache Research Group

The first meeting of the Research Group on Migraine and Headache was held in London in 1969. It was a very successful round-the-table 'think session' which led to a series of definitions, which were promulgated, on an international scale. The Research Group had a close collaboration with the British Migraine Trust, which led to international conferences on migraine and headache. This Research Group has been very active, and Stephen D. Silberstein (Philadelphia, USA) is the present chair (2011).

Motor Neuron Diseases Research Group

The Research Group on Motor Neuron Diseases was founded in 1972 and Michael Swash was an active promoter. The group is sponsoring its own journal, *Amyotrophic Lateral Sclerosis and Related Motor Neuron Disorders.*

It is playing a major role in the planning and contribution to the annual symposium on MND/ALS organized by the Motor Neuron Disease Association

(UK). Albert Ludolph (Ulm, Germany) is the present Chair and Orla Hardiman (Dublin, Ireland) Co-Chair.

Multiple Sclerosis Research Group

The WFN Research Group on Multiple Sclerosis was first a WFN Research Group with Torben Fog (Copenhagen, Denmark) as an active and hard-working Chairman. The development in MS research led to the establishment of the International Federation of Multiple Sclerosis Societies, publishing bi-monthly abstracts of all international meetings related to multiple sclerosis, and the two groups merged. Since the International Federation of Multiple Sclerosis Societies had its focus more on practical objectives such as making the public and the health authorities better acquainted with the disease and also of raising funds to help sufferers, in 1977 Torben Fog regarded it necessary to have a separate existence of the two organizations. The International Federation of Multiple Sclerosis Societies is represented on the Research Committee of the WFN as corporate membership.

The Multiple Sclerosis International Federation has, in collaboration with the WHO, gathered data from 112 countries on the epidemiology of MS and the availability and accessibility of resources to diagnose, inform, treat, support, and rehabilitate people with MS worldwide. The Atlas of MS raises awareness and encourages exploration of the validity and robustness of existing data on epidemiology and services available to people with MS.

There are specific MS research programmes and fellowships, such as the Du Pré Grants (which allow researchers to travel to MS centers of excellence), the McDonald Fellowship, the Charcot Award (lifetime achievement award) and International Research Meeting Grants (aid towards international research meetings).

The International Pediatric MS Study Group (IPMSSG) facilitates and coordinates activities of the group and provides and secures funding for their research meetings.

Neuroethics Research Group

Franz Gerstenbrand (Vienna, Austria) is the present Chair (2011). This was previously a standing Committee of the WFN, but was then transferred to a Research Group.

Research Group on Neuro-Rehabilitation and Restorative Neurology

The Research Group on Neurological Rehabilitation was first established as a Problem Commission in 1963. It was planned as one group with a Secretariat in the west and another group having their secretariat in the east, preferably in Prague, under the supervision of Dr Obrda in Professor Kamil Henner's service (16).

In 1964 there was a founding meeting of the WFN Problem Commission of Rehabilitation and Physical Medicine in Neurology for the eastern hemisphere. The principles of rehabilitation were discussed, and there was agreement that:

1 There should be a rehabilitation department in every hospital for acute cases, as well as for those who have been discharged from hospital care.

2 There should be special sections in hospitals for each particular type of illness. The same is true of larger neurological centres.

3 There should be re-educational dispensaries distributed throughout the district.

4 There should be special centres for those patients who need more prolonged care, which should be orientated towards social and occupational aspects. They should be located near the big hospitals, as they require consultations with other branches of medicine.

The scientific activities of WFN rehabilitation research were mainly concerned with rehabilitation of sufferers from cerebral vascular disease and from head injury. A symposium on rehabilitation after head injury was held in Gothenburg in 1971. In 1976, it was divided into three subgroups, one for eastern Europe, one for western Europe, and one for Scandinavia and other European countries. Because of the particular relevance of neurological rehabilitation to developing countries, the secretaries of this group were also prepared to advise the WHO on rehabilitation.

The name of the group was later expanded to the Research Group on Neurorehabilitation and Restorative Neurology. The present chair (2011) is Jorgen Borg, Uppsala, Sweden.

The World Federation for Neuro-rehabilitation was formed during the 3rd World Congress on Neurological Rehabilitation in Venice in 2002. The aim of the organization is to promote the cause of neurological rehabilitation on a worldwide basis, mainly through organizing a congress every three years. Professor Michael Barnes (Newcastle upon Tyne, UK) was elected first President of the new Federation. The relationship to the WFN Research Group has not been clarified.

Research Group on Neurosonology

Diagnostic ultrasound has become an important tool in clinical neurology. The Research Group on Neurosonology, previously Ultrasonics in Neurology, is a very active group that has organized Advanced Teaching Courses in close

THE WORLD FEDERATION OF NEUROLOGY APPLIED RESEARCH COMMITTEE | **133**

relation with the World Congresses. It is one of the few Research Groups that has instituted a specific research project—'Neurosonology in Acute Ischaemic Stroke'. The Chair is Manfred Kaps, Giessen, Germany.

Research Group on Organization and Delivery of Care

This group was established in New Delhi in 1989. The initiative came from Bosko Barac and Jagjit S. Chopra. Bosco Barac served as Chairman until 2009 (see 'The Continuing Education Committee', p. 100).

Research Group on Palliative Care

The WFN Research Committee decided in 2000 that there is a need for better management of patients with progressive and incurable neurological disorders, particularly at the end of life. A Research Group was established to provide a forum for exchange of experience, to initiate and coordinate research projects, help formulate guidelines, and improve training and education of neurologists in the field of palliative care. The present Chair (2011) is Raymond Voltz, Köln, Germany.

Research Group on Parkinsonism and Related Disorders (formerly Research Group on Extrapyramidal Diseases)

This is one of the most active Research Groups of the WFN. Melvin Yahr was the founder and led it with distinction for many years until Donald Calne took over in 2001. The WFN established a lectureship to honour the contributions of Dr Yahr. In 1987, the Research Committee met during the annual AAN meeting in New York and re-established its policy on the sponsorship of symposia and also discussed travel fellowship.

In 1969 it was discussed whether the Research Committee on Industrial and Environmental Neurology should sponsor the establishment of a new Research Group on Parkinsonism, but it was agreed after discussion to defer this suggestion.

The Research Group on Parkinsonism and Related Disorders (RG-PRD) is represented on the WFN's Research Committee and advises it in matters concerning Parkinson's disease and other movement disorders. Its mission is to foster, encourage, and support the development and advancement of neurological scientific investigation related to Parkinson's disease and other movement disorders.

Another important mission is to promote knowledge about available treatment options and strategies for Parkinson's disease and other movement disorders. The official publication of the Research Group is the journal *Parkinsonism and Related Disorders.* In Amsterdam in 2007, Erik Wolters was elected new Chair, replacing Donald Calne.

Research Group on Sleep

Sleep problems are important. As well as causing distress to the individual, sleep problems also create a significant burden on society. Sleep apnoea, restless legs syndrome, and psychophysiological insomnia are among the most common alterations to sleep. Poor quality of sleep or insufficient sleep can also have a negative effect on the health of an individual. Sleep deprivation has been associated with a decline in mental health.

However, most sleep disorders are preventable or treatable, yet less than a third of sufferers seek professional help.

World Sleep Day aims to reduce the burden of sleep disorders on society by encouraging better understanding of sleep conditions and calling for more research into sleep medicine and treatment.

The present Chair (2011) is Antonio Culebras (Syracuse, New York, USA).

Research Group on Space and Underwater Neurology

The present Chair (2011) is Franz Gerstenbrand (Vienna, Austria).

Research Group on Cerebral Circulation

This group was renamed the Research Group on Cerebrovascular Disease in 1979.

Professor Klaus Zülch retired in 1979 from the position as the Secretary of the group. David Klein, who was the Research Committee Secretary Treasurer, transferred $10,665.65 to the WFN in 1987. A major activity of the group was that of sponsoring the biennial Salzburg Conference on Cerebral Vascular Disease.

An international board of charter members, including H. Lechner, F. Gotoh, JS Meyer, C. Loeb, C. Fazio, J. Marshall, and A. Agnoli, organized the Salzburg Conference. The first Salzburg Conference on Cerebrovascular Disease (SCCVD) was held in 1962. Salzburg was the hometown of Christian Doppler, the founder of a concept later developed for ultrasound cerebral flow measurements. The SCCVD was designed to provide a platform for the exchange of new research information on cerebrovascular diseases.

The activity of the Salzburg Conference group also involved closer contact with the WFN Research Group. It was agreed that all 400 individuals registered with that conference should be invited to become members of the Research Group. It was involved in organizing international symposia, and its activities became gradually so central to neurosciences that international stroke organizations have developed. Helmut Lechner, Carlo Loeb, John Marshall, and John Stirling Meyer were all chairmen in 1982.

It was suggested that the journal *Stroke* should become the official journal of the WFN Research Group on Cerebrovascular Disorders.

The Research Group on Cerebrovascular Disease has not been disbanded. Cerebrovascular disorders are central to neurology, and the WFN therefore decided to establish a separate Stroke Affairs Committee to act at the interface between the ISS and other stroke associations around the world (17,18).

Research Group on Neuroimmunology and Neurovirology

Neuroimmunology emerged among the neurosciences in the 1970s, and the first International Congress of Neuroimmunology was held in Stresa, Italy, in 1982. A WFN Research Group on Neuroimmunology was founded in 1981, and the *Journal of Neuroimmunology* became the official journal. The Second International Congress of Neuroimmunology was held in Philadelphia, PA, in 1987. It was then decided to start the International Society of Neuroimmunology, which became an independent society.

The International Society of Neurovirology was established under the leadership of Kamel Khalili. This was independent of the WFN but with many members of the old WFN Research Group taking part. Development of both of these organizations has been a smooth transition, and large international organizations have evolved incorporating many basic scientists among the clinicians.

The two Research Groups met during the World Congress of Neurology in Hamburg in 1986 and decided to merge the two groups, with Richard Johnson as the Chair of the new Research Group. Neuroimmunology and neurovirology saw a dramatic expansion in the following years, including the non-clinical aspects. The Research Groups do not exist as WFN Research Groups today.

There is not a Research Committee on epilepsy. The International League Against Epilepsy (ILAE) is much older than the World Federation of Neurology. Epilepsy is a major element of clinical neurology and the cooperation between the WFN and ILAE is strong. At the meeting of the WFN Steering Committee in 1982, it was suggested that epilepsy research should be an important element of the WFN.

The Research Group on Neurotraumatology

Professor Nenad Gracevic (Zagreb) was an active chairman for a long period. Cervos-Navarro took over in New Delhi 1989. The group was later disbanded.

The Research Group on Cerebrospinal Fluid

It was reorganized by A. Lowenthal, but was later disbanded.

The International Federation of Societies for EEG and Clinical Neurophysiology (IFSECN)

This is an interdisciplinary society established as early as 1947, before the WFN was founded. They sponsored two quadrennial international congresses—The Congress on Clinical Neurophysiology, and The Congress on EMG and Related Clinical Neurophysiology. In 2003, it was decided to discontinue having two separate International Congresses, and the two were then consolidated into one quadrennial comprehensive congress.

Behavioral Neurology International

Behavioral Neurology International is an interdisciplinary society of behavioural scientists including neurologists, psychiatrists, and psychologists concerned with human behaviour and behavioural disorders. When Sidney Walton III was President, they decided to apply for membership as a Research Group of the WFN Research Committee. In 1987, the Research Committee accepted corporate membership of the organization, since it already was an established international organization.

New WFN Research Committee Guidelines

In 2000, the new WFN Research Committee evaluated new guidelines for the Research Groups and accepted the following (19):

1 Each RG [Research Group] will elect its own Chair and officers for a four-year renewable term.

2 Each RG will determine its own mission, consistent with the goals and objectives of the WFN.

3 A yearly progress and financial report will be provided to the WFN Secretariat.

4 All international meetings and conferences organized by the RG must be approved by the WFN Trustees on the recommendation of the WFN Education Committee.

5 The publication of official RG journals must be coordinated with the WFN Publications Committee.

THE WORLD FEDERATION OF NEUROLOGY APPLIED RESEARCH COMMITTEE | **137**

6 The membership of an RG is open to all qualified neurologists and neuroscientists. If a qualified individual is denied membership an appeal can be made to the Research Committee or Trustees.

7 New Research Groups may be admitted to the WFN upon suitable application to the Secretariat and approval by the Research Committee and Trustees. The application should contain a mission statement, strategies by which the mission will be accomplished, membership list and officers.

8 Funds raised by any RG are WFN funds and are subject to UK Charity Commission regulations. Disbursement of such funds must be in furtherance of the WFN's stated charitable objectives.

9 Research Groups may be disassociated from the WFN for just cause by a majority vote of the Research Committee and confirmation of this action by the Trustees.

References

1 **Poser CM.** The World Federation of Neurology: the formative period 1955–1961. *J Neur Sci* 1993; **120**: 218–27.

2 **Van Bogaert L.** Presidential Report. *J Neur Sci* 1966; **3**: 439–50.

3 **Minutes of the Meeting of the Council of Delegates, Amsterdam 1975.** *J Neur Sci* 1976; **29**: 427–36.

4 **WFN Research Committee, Amsterdam, 10 September 1977.** *J Neur Sci* 1978; **36**: 303–8.

5 **Third World Medical Research Foundation Makes Grant.** *World Neurol* 1987; 2(3): 1.

6 **Walton J.** The Statutes of the Research Committee of the World Federation of Neurology. *J Neur Sci* 1979; **43**: 490–3.

7 **Walton J.** Report of the Chairman of the Research Committee. *World Neurol* 1986; **1**(2): 1–2.

8 **Cotzias GC, Van Woert MH, Schiffer LM.** Aromatic amino acids and modification of Parkinsonism. *N Engl J Med* 1967; **276**: 374–9.

9 **Kurland LT.** Report on the Activities of the WFN Problem Commission on Geographic Neurology, Statistics and Epidemiology. *J Neur Sci* 1964; **1**: 485–90.

10 **Kurland LT, Hyllested K.** Synopsis of the third conference of geographical neurology. *J Neur Sci* 1964; **1**: 488–90.

11 **Lowenthal A.** Report on the activities of the WFN Problem Commission on Neurochemistry. *J Neur Sci* 1964; **1**: 298.

12 **Walton J.** WFN Research Committee Research Group on Neuromuscular Diseases. *J Neur Sci* 1970; **10**: 504–16.

13 **Stephan H.** Report of the activities of the WFN Problem Commission on Neuroanatomy. *J Neur Sci* 1964; **1**: 199–200.

14 **Franceschetti A.** Report of the activities of the WFN Problem Commission on Neuro-Ophthalmology (Eastern Hemisphere). *J Neur Sci* 1964; **1**: 197–8.

15 **Newell FW.** Report of the activities of the WFN Problem Commission on Neuro-Ophthalmology (Western Hemisphere). *J Neur Sci* 1964; **1**: 197.

16 **Obrda K.** Minutes of the Founding Meeting of the WFN Problem Commission on Rehabilitation and Physical Medicine in Neurology, for the Eastern Hemisphere (Prague, 10 October 1964). *J Neurol Sci* 1965; **2**: 575–80.

17 **Lechner H, Meyer JS.** The SCCVD: Past and Future. *World Neurol* 1998; **13**(2): 6.

18 **Bogousslavsky J, Aarli J, Kimura J.** Stroke and neurology: a plea from the WFN. *Lancet Neurol* 2003; **2**(4): 212–3.

19 **Munsat T.** Report of the Research Committee. *World Neurol* 2001; **16**(1): 8.

Chapter 5

Communication in the World Federation of Neurology

World Neurology 1960–1962

In 1959 the WFN decided it should sponsor its own scientific journal. *World Neurology* was the journal, and the first issue was published July 1960. It published articles in English, French, German, or Spanish, with summaries in the other three languages. It also included a newsletter similar to that which Pearce Bailey had started for *Neurology*.

The Problem Commissions (later renamed the Research Groups) were at that time already established elements of the WFN. The new journal was to serve as a forum for the Problem Commissions, with announcements of their meetings and reports from national and international meetings in neurology. Each issue should contain at least one review article written upon request by an authority on the subject (1).

Charles Poser became the first Editor-in-Chief, with Ludo van Bogaert and Pearce Bailey Associate Editors. A total of 2300 paid subscriptions were recorded once it became known, but the numbers were very slow to increase. Conflicts appeared. Charles Poser was replaced with Gilbert Glaser as Editor-in-Chief in September 1961 and *World Neurology* stopped publication in December 1962. The history of the brief life of the first *World Neurology* is described in Chapter 2.

Journal of the Neurological Sciences

Ludo van Bogaert and Armand Lowenthal then negotiated a contract with Elsevier, and a new journal, *Journal of the Neurological Sciences*, the official Bulletin of the World Federation of Neurology, was born in 1964, with six issues a year. Macdonald Critchley was the first Editor-in-Chief. When Critchley became WFN President in 1965, John Walton was appointed his successor, and he remained Editor-in-Chief until 1977. Gilbert Glaser was the Regional Editor for North America, Oscar Trelles for South America, Ludo van Bogaert for Europe, and Graeme Robertson for the Far East.

John Walton put his mark upon the new journal. It became first and foremost a scientific journal, but each volume also contained information from the WFN. The Secretary-Treasurer General contributed with minutes from the meetings of the Council of Delegates. The Editors-in-Chief described the annual progress of the two scientific journals, the *Journal of the Neurological Sciences* and *Acta Neuropathologica*. From 1967, the Research Committee reported regularly about the activities of the Research Groups. The journal also published announcements of international meetings in neurology.

During these years, there was a slow but steady increase in the circulation of the journal. The size of each issue was doubled in 1967. In 1969, Elsevier concluded that a minimum of 900 subscriptions should be sold annually, and preferably about 1000 in order to cover completely the entire cost of publishing and advertising the journal. The company was, however, prepared to continue to publish the journal indefinitely because of the potential for further expansion.

The *Journal of the Neurological Sciences* was self-supporting and did not receive any subsidies from the WFN (2). The submission rate increased from 93 in 1968 (eight rejected) to 155 in 1972 (44 rejected). The leading countries for submissions were the UK, USA, the Netherlands, Canada, Belgium, and Japan. The total annual circulation of the journal was about 1000. The subscription rate increased from 521 in 1964 to 930 in 1972. In 1973, the Editor-in-Chief requested an increase in the grant towards secretarial expenses, namely from £250 to £500. The grant was for the Editor's secretarial and postage expenses only. Without this aid from the WFN, the Editor-in-Chief, John Walton, was not willing to continue as editor.

Succeeding John Walton, Bryan Matthews of Oxford became Editor-in-Chief in 1977. The next Editor-in-Chief was George Bruyn of Amsterdam, who was succeeded by James Toole of Winston-Salem in 1989. Toole became President of the WFN in 1997, and Robert P. Lisak of Detroit took over as the Editor-in-Chief in 1998. Richard A. Lewis and Paula Dore-Duffy have been Deputy Directors; the administrator and supporting editor is Susan E. Hutton.

During this 13-year period, the journal has showed considerable growth and improved its impact throughout the medical world. The submission rate soared annually from 400 to 1325. The initial increase may relate to the journal going electronic, but the continuing increase probably relates to an increased stature, which is seen in the impact factor. The impact factor (reflecting the average number of citations over the two preceding years) rose from 1.84 to 2.359, and the journal now ranks 68th of all 156 journals in Thomson Reuters' clinical neurology category. These indicators are a reflection of the journal's growing importance as an international journal covering all aspects of neurology (3).

The implementation in May 2006 of the Elsevier Editorial System, online submission/review process software, has acted as a catalyst for this growth. The evolution of the journal continues to be reflected in the changing dynamics of authors and ad hoc reviewers.

The five leading countries for submissions remain Japan, China, the USA, South Korea, and Italy. However, submissions from regions including Africa, Egypt, Iran, Jordan, Lebanon, Palestine, Qatar, the Russian Federation, and Saudi Arabia demonstrate the growing global impact on emerging markets.

Special issues and supplements have become a regular feature of the journal. During 2009–2010, guest editors have produced one supplement and two special issues dedicated to multiple sclerosis research and another special issue featured vascular dementia: Franz Fazekas of Graz Medical University, Austria, and Bernd C. Kieseier of Heinrich Heine University, Düsseldorf, Germany, produced the supplement, 'Translating New Insights Into Treatment in Multiple Sclerosis', Robert Zivadinov of the State University of New York at Buffalo and Alireza Minagar of Louisiana State University Health Sciences Center, Shreveport, focused on a special issue titled, 'Evidence for Gray Matter Pathology in Multiple Sclerosis: A Neuroimaging Approach', Amos D. Korczyn, Natan M. Bornstein, and Laszlo Vecsei, all from Tel-Aviv Sourasky Medical Center, Israel, edited the special issue, 'Vascular Dementia Proceedings of the Fifth International Congress on Vascular Diseases'. Otto R. Hommes, chairman of the European Charcot Foundation, and Mieke Friedrichs, managing director of the foundation, presented another special issue, 'Multiple Sclerosis and Gender'.

Elsevier owns the journal, and the present contract for the *Journal of the Neurological Sciences* runs until 2015.

The newsletter of the World Federation of Neurology— *World Neurology*

Armand Lowenthal realized the need for an EFNS newsletter, and tried to create a *Bulletin of Information*, which would present news from the Problem Commissions (Research Groups), and be distributed to all neurologists of the WFN. It proved difficult to collect enough information, and for several years, the *Journal of the Neurological Sciences* served as the only WFN newsletter with regular announcements and minutes from committee meetings. It was, however, difficult to combine the newsletter function with that of a scientific journal.

When Richard Masland became the WFN President in 1981, he realized that the organization needed its own newsletter. Together with the Secretary-Treasurer General, James Toole, sufficient commercial sponsorship was obtained. The new newsletter, *World Neurology*, was published on 15 November 1983. Considering its function, the name was appropriate, but it had nothing to do with the previous WFN-owned periodical. Only the name was the same.

The first four issues were circulated to over 18 000 neurologists throughout the world. The management group of the coming WFN World Congress of Neurology to be held in Hamburg covered the costs. They were related to the upcoming congress in 1985. Issues 2 and 3 were published in 1984, and accompanied by the announcements for the Congress, while issue 4 was the Pre-Congress issue.

The main contents of the first issue were highlights of the Meeting of the Council of Delegates and the Research Committee Hamburg, 10–11 June 1983, two years before the Congress. After that, the cost of publishing and distributing the newsletter had to be met by the WFN.

The WFN Secretary-Treasurer General, James Toole, had the newsletter produced, printed and circulated from Winston-Salem. The publishing and distribution of *World Neurology* to neurologists worldwide was first made possible by an educational grant from the Parke Davis Division of the Warner-Lambert Company, then Eldred Smith-Gordon, and subsequently with Cambridge Medical Publications.

From 1986, Raven Press printed *World Neurology* quarterly. The first issue in 1986 was published as Volume 1, Number 1. The newsletter was now printed on glossy paper and had WFN President Richard Masland's Report of the Hamburg Conference on the front page. It soon had a worldwide distribution of over 20 000 and fulfilled its function as the mouthpiece of the WFN with information about future congresses and symposia, as well as presentations from various neurology centres around the world.

Frank Clifford Rose was elected WFN Secretary-Treasurer General in 1989. In 1990, he became the first Editor-in-Chief of *World Neurology*. Robert B. Daroff and James Toole were Co-Editors. The newsletter now changed its appearance. Number 1, Volume 5, had 16 pages, which became the set standard for the next 15 years. Its unique importance is that for a long time it was the sole force that united the whole of the WFN, since every member of the Federation received a copy. Since then, each issue of *World Neurology* has had a special President's Column with direct communication from the leader of the federation.

Frank Clifford Rose was the Editor-in-Chief during the most constructive modernization phase in the history of the WFN. It lasted during Walton and

COMMUNICATION IN THE WORLD FEDERATION OF NEUROLOGY | **143**

Toole's Presidencies, and some of the last elements of the re-organization were first put in place during Kimura's Presidency. Rose took care to involve the readers in the modernization process and was concerned that all WFN members were informed about the process.

Another special feature during Rose's period as the Editor-in-Chief was the publishing of news and information about planning of future World Congresses of Neurology, especially Vancouver 1993 and Buenos Aires 1997, and to some extent also London 2001, which took place during and immediately following his editorial period.

When James Toole succeeded John Walton as WFN President, Frank Clifford Rose retired as Editor-in-Chief of *World Neurology*, and the WFN Publications Committee chose Jagjit S. Chopra of Chandigarh (India) as the new Editor. He had been the Secretary-General of the very successful World Congress of Neurology in New Delhi in 1989. Chopra printed and distributed the newspaper from India at great savings to the organization. At this time, Elsevier contracted with the WFN to produce the newsletter and solicit appropriate advertisements.

Chopra's well-written editorials reviewed the contents of each article of the issue, putting them into a global perspective with the background of his deep insight into how the WFN works and his knowledge of modern clinical neurosciences. The improved layout settings facilitated easier reading. Fonts were more legible, and the spacing improved so the newsletter was easier to read. Chopra was also the newsletter's photographer, and each issue of *World Neurology* successfully presented WFN attendance at business meetings of the WFN as well as important regional meetings. Chopra reported from several regional neurology meetings, and supplied them with new and colourful illustrations. *World Neurology* also presented annual reports from the main WFN Committees. Like Rose, Chopra took care to include information about the structural changes taking place in the organization.

The new President, James Toole, organized the important Ad-hoc Strategic Planning group meeting at Sopwell House Hotel at St Albans in 1999. At this meeting, the WFN national delegates met and discussed the structure of the Federation after ten years of constructive reorganization. Chopra covered the meeting well, and the subsequent issue of *World Neurology* set out detailed information about the changes now planned for the organization.

In 2008, Mark Hallett became the next Editor-in-Chief. He included more information about the national neurological societies, and introduced the 'Profiles in Neurology' series and the clinically exciting 'Neurological Pearls'. The size of the journal increased, and the number of issues per year increased to six. The increased volume also brought more important scientific communication such as 'Highlights from the *Journal of the Neurological Sciences*'.

144 THE HISTORY OF THE WORLD FEDERATION OF NEUROLOGY

Hallett has also been very active in bringing reports from international and regional meetings. Like Rose and Chopra before him, Hallett publishes updated information about the internal life and development of the organization. At the same time, *World Neurology* has become more extrovert, bringing information about the contemporary development in neurology to a global level.

Johan Aarli succeeded Mark Hallett as Editor-in-Chief in 2012. At the same time, the digital revolution, with advanced websites and transfer from print to digital editions, and the change of ownership complicated the process, which is not yet finished (September 2012).

The WFN on the website

During Kimura's Presidency, the WFN started to explore the use of a website and online newsletter in addition to the official publications, *the Journal of the Neurological Sciences* and *World Neurology*, which then represented the official WFN documents.

The website itself has undergone a radical transformation and has become more informative and interactive. Developing the WFN website has been a long process. An interactive website requires close collaboration with the WFN staff, which at first was difficult with the present capacity. The website structure then became a reality, and it is now easy to find on the WFN home pages on the Internet.

The revised website (www.worldneurologyonline.com) was launched at the World Neurology Congress in Marrakesh in November 2011. The contents are as follows: About Us, Education, Global Networks, Publications, Members Societies, Meetings and Congresses, and Social Networks.

Acta Neuropathologica

With Franz Seitelberger as Editor-In-Chief, *Acta Neuropathologica* was for a period the official journal of three of the WFN Research Groups: neuropathology, comparative neuropathology, and comparative neuroanatomy.

During the board discussion in 1973, Franz Seitelberger pointed out that *Acta Neuropathologica* received no aid from the WFN, and that he would be unable to carry on as Editor without it. There were, however, voices from the floor that since the Council had just approved a 100% increase in membership fees, some national societies would not endorse the continued subsidy to the two journals. At a show of hands, only one member voted against the WFN continuing to give a grant to the Editors for secretarial expenses. The remainder of the members who voted were in favour of supporting the extra expenses. Since then, an International Society of Neuropathology has been established and

COMMUNICATION IN THE WORLD FEDERATION OF NEUROLOGY | **145**

become affiliated with the WFN as a Corporate Member, but the Research Group on Neuropathology remains in the WFN.

The financial crisis persisted into the 1980s, and it was decided that all publications sponsored by the WFN should be self-supporting, starting with scrutinizing the contracts of the *Journal of the Neurological Sciences, Acta Neuropathologica*, and the WFN *World Neurology* newsletter. The WFN-Finance Committee recommended that the annual subsidy to *Acta Neuropathologica* be discontinued by 1 January 1988.

WFN Seminars in Clinical Neurology

Chairman of the WFN Education Committee Ted Munsat initiated a series of pilot studies using the AAN programme *Continuum: Lifelong Learning in Neurology*. A major strategic aim of that programme, which started in 2001, was to develop and promote affordable and effective continuing neurological education for neurologists and related healthcare providers. The programme is modelled on the American Academy of Neurology's highly successful 'Continuum' and includes case-oriented information, key points, multiple choice questions, annotated references, and abundant use of graphic material. The publications were published by Demos Medical Publishing. Dr Jerome Engel is series editor. Funding for the programme was provided by unrestricted educational grants.

The first publication included the neglected field of neuro-urology and neurological bowel dysfunction, and was followed by epilepsy, global issues for the practising neurologist, dystonia, stroke, and multiple sclerosis for the practising neurologist, and neurological consequences of malnutrition.

The WFN CME programme offers the provision of neurological educational material. To date there are forty-three countries participating in the programme. Through this training neurological teams globally have enhanced their skills as well as being made aware of new techniques, best practices, and treatments.

Teleconferences

When the WFN was born, in 1957, it was not possible, within reasonable economic limits, for a global leadership to convene at regular intervals. Postal communication was essential. Modern telecommunication has had a dramatic effect, and teleconferences became a regular communication event during James Toole's Presidency. We have tried to make the minutes from the teleconferences available online, but the practical consequences are not compatible with the accessibility and the speed needed.

References

1 **Poser CM.** The World Federation of Neurology: the formative period 1955–1961. Personal recollections. *J Neur Sci* 1993; **120**: 218–27.

2 **Walton J.** Editor's Report of the Journal of the Neurological Sciences. Barcelona 1973. *J Neur Sci* 1974; **21**: 502–5.

3 **Lisak RP.** JNS continues along its path of growth and expansion. *World Neurol* 2010; **25**: 15.

Chapter 6

Regional Neurological Associations

In most countries, neurology as a clinical specialty was established many years before the birth of the World Federation of Neurology (WFN). This chapter deals with the differences in the regional organization of the WFN. They have little or nothing to do with the degree of specialization in medicine and the development of hospitals, but more with the abilities of the WFN to establish a worldwide network of neurologists. The WFN regional neurological associations are different from each other, partly because of history, and partly because of the complexity of other medical institutions in the region.

When the WFN was conceived, van Bogaert had three major regional associations in his mind: the Greater European, the Greater American, and the Greater Asian-Oceanian. Today, the WFN comprises six regional associations, each with a different history and background.

What is a 'qualified neurologist'?

The WFN is a global federation. Each national neurological society is an individual unit of the WFN. Each neurologist is a member of his/her national neurological society. Some societies, such as the American Academy of Neurology (AAN), the Brazilian, the German, and the Japanese, are big. Others are very small, for example some African and European national societies.

A national neurological society can be established if there are five or more 'qualified neurologists' resident in a country that does not already have a member society.

What is a 'qualified neurologist'? The definition is not clear, and is not necessarily based upon traditional western criteria of the specialty. It is also dependent upon the geographic setting, the differences in the spectrum of health challenges of the nation, and the definitions of clinical specialties. This was clearly described by Noshir Wadia, who wrote 'The main task of Indian neurologists has been, rightly to identify and document the prevalence of local diseases, as seen by them and through research, to build up a neurological nosography pertinent to our country' (1).

When a national neurological society is established, it has to be recommended by the Trustees and approved at a meeting of the Council of Delegates, who are presented with the total medical situation. Today (2011) 113 national neurological societies are members of the WFN.

The WFN regions

The WFN regions are crucial in the discussions on the structure of the WFN. Regional Vice Presidents have been elected since 1965. Until 2001, the Council of Delegates elected them, without their function being defined. Nor did they represent the respective regional neurological associations—except in their function as editorial board of *World Neurology*.

When Johan Aarli was elected First Vice President in 2001, he initiated a discussion on the relationship between the WFN central administration and the Regional Vice Presidents. By 2003, the Trustees had arrived at a new definition of the Regional Vice Presidents, which was approved by the WFN Council of Delegates at the World Congress in Sydney. The discussions at the Council of Delegates 2003 made it clear that the Regional Vice Presidents would have a stronger basis when representing a regional neurological association. No changes were introduced, as the current Regional Vice Presidents were then mid-way through the terms of their office. The WFN did, however, prefer the term Regional Director and not Regional Vice President. This also involved definitions of the regions, and the WFN decided to follow the structure of the World Health Organization (WHO).

The WHO is the directing and coordinating authority for health within the United Nations. The WFN has a close collaboration with the WHO, which is responsible for providing leadership on global health matters and shaping the health research agenda. It is important for the WFN with its geographical and regional programmes to operate within the WHO geography.

Members of the WHO are grouped according to regional distribution in six WHO regions, the African region, the American region, the South-East Asian region, the European region, the East Mediterranean region, and the Western Pacific region. Each WHO region has a regional office, in Brazzaville, Congo, for the African region, in New Delhi, India, for the South-East Asian region, in Washington, DC, for the American region, in Copenhagen, Denmark, for the European region, in Cairo, Egypt, for the Eastern Mediterranean region, and in Manila, Philippines for the Western Pacific region.

Since neurology is so well developed in the Americas, and also for linguistic reasons, the WFN has found it practical to have one North American and one Latin American region, and, in agreement with the Asian-Oceanian Association of Neurology, only one Asian-Oceanian Region of Neurology.

The WHO structure was drawn up in 1948, and is based upon political, social, economic, and other decisions that are still relevant in 2011. The WHO African region comprises 46 Member States: Algeria, Angola, Benin, Botswana, Burkina Faso, Burundi, Cameroon, Cape Verde, Central African Republic, Chad, Comoros, Congo, Cote d'Ivoire, Democratic Republic of Congo, Equatorial Guinea, Eritrea, Ethiopia, Gabon, Gambia, Ghana, Guinea, Guinea-Bissau, Kenya, Lesotho, Liberia, Madagascar, Malawi, Mali, Mauritania, Mauritius, Mozambique, Namibia, Niger, Nigeria, Rwanda, São Tomé & Príncipe, Senegal, Seychelles, Sierra Leone, South Africa, Swaziland, Tanzania, Togo, Uganda, Zambia, and Zimbabwe.

According to the WHO structure, Algeria is a part of the WHO African and not of the Eastern Mediterranean region, while Morocco, Tunisia, Libya, Egypt, Eritrea, Sudan, and Somalia are outside the WHO African Region.

The WHO Eastern Mediterranean region comprises the following national states: Afghanistan, Bahrain, Djibouti, Egypt, Arab Republic of Iran, Iraq, Jordan, Kuwait, Lebanon, Libya, Morocco, Oman, Pakistan, Palestine, Qatar, Saudi Arabia, Somalia, Sudan, Syrian Arab Republic, Tunisia, United Arab Emirates, and Yemen.

The WHO South-East Asia region comprises 11 national states: Bangladesh, Bhutan, Democratic People's Republic of Korea, India, Indonesia, Maldives, Myanmar, Nepal, Sri Lanka, Thailand, and Timor Leste.

The WHO Western Pacific Region is huge, with approximately 1.6 billion inhabitants and nearly one-third of the world's population: American Samoa, Australia, Brunei, Cambodia, China, Cook Islands, Fiji, French Polynesia, Guam, Hong Kong, Japan, Kiribati, Lao People's Democratic Republic, Macao, Malaysia, Micronesia, Mongolia, Nauru, New Caledonia, New Zealand, Niue, Northern Mariana Islands, Palau, Papua, Philippines, Pitcairn Island, Republic of Korea, Samoa, Singapore, Solomon Island, Tokelau, Tonga, Tuvalo, Vanuatu, Viet Nam, Wallis & Fortuna.

The WHO region of the Americas comprises Anguilla, Antigua and Barbuda, Argentina, Aruba, Bahamas, Barbados, Belize, Bermuda, Bolivia, Brazil, British Virgin Islands, Canada, Cayman Islands, Chile, Columbia, Costa Rica, Cuba, Dominica, Dominican Republic, El Salvador, Ecuador, US/Mexican Border, French Guiana, Grenada, Guadeloupe, Guatemala, Guyana, Haiti, Honduras, Jamaica, Martinique, Mexico, Montserrat, Netherlands Antilles, Nicaragua, Panama, Paraguay, Peru, Puerto Rico, Saint Kitts and Nevis, Saint Lucia, Saint Vincent and the Grenadines, Suriname, Trinidad & Tobago, Turks & Caicos Islands, Uruguay, Venezuela, USA.

The WHO European region comprises Albania, Andorra, Armenia, Austria, Azerbaijan, Belarus, Belgium, Bosnia and Herzegovina, Bulgaria, Croatia,

Cyprus, Czech Republic, Denmark, Estonia, Finland, France, Georgia, Germany, Hungary, Iceland, Ireland, Israel, Italy, Kazakhstan, Kyrgyzstan, Latvia, Lithuania, Luxembourg, Malta, Monaco, Montenegro, Netherlands, Norway, Poland, Portugal, Republic of Moldova, Romania, Russian Federation, San Marino, Serbia, Slovakia, Slovenia, Spain, Sweden, Switzerland, Tajikistan, the former Yugoslav Republic of Macedonia, Turkey, Turkmenistan, Ukraine, United Kingdom of Great Britain and Northern Ireland, Uzbekistan.

The WFN and the American Academy of Neurology

The American Association of Neurology was founded in 1875. The major international neurological association is the AAN, which was founded in 1947. The AAN has considerable international memberships and operates in the important field of international commitment.

Houston Merritt was one of the strongest supporters for forming the institution (2). At the meeting of the AAN in 1956, Houston Merritt and Pearce Bailey proposed the creation of a world neurological federation. The proposal was approved unanimously. According to Poser, van Bogaert and his European colleagues had viewed the discipline of neurology as a rather cosy, loosely organized association based on continuous close personal friendship (3). There can be no doubt that the two American neurologists influenced the WFN constitution with their background and experiences from an already well-established neurological organization. A truly international cooperation now took hold, in large part owing to their persuasion.

The AAN and the Canadian Neurological Sciences Federation (a Canadian umbrella organization representing neurology, neurosurgery, clinical neurophysiology, and child neurology) are English speaking, while the remaining countries in the Americas are primarily Spanish or Portuguese speaking.

A decentralization process—without Africa

Many national neurological societies are members of a regional neurological association. They comprise the Asian Oceanian Association of Neurology (AOAN), the Pan American Association of Neurology, the North American Association of Neurology, the European Federation of Neurological Societies (EFNS), the Pan African Association of Neurological Sciences (PAANS) and the Pan Arab Union of Neurological Societies (PAUNS).

In order to understand the present structure, which will certainly be modified during the coming years, we have to start with the formative period. At that time, the decentralization process was the key issue. How could the WFN become a global organization?

The first President of the WFN, Ludo van Bogaert, realized the importance of the WFN as a global organization. This is inevitable today, but was not without problems in 1957. Van Bogaert proposed the decentralization plan as early as 1962 (4). The plan had three aspects: a more equitable division of labour among the WFN member societies, a greater sense of participation in the total programme by the individual member societies, and a more equitable distribution of financial responsibility for the support of the WFN programme. This plan was presented at a time when the financial crisis of the WFN was the dominating problem (4). But the most important consequence of the plan proved to be the regional organizations. In turn, they served as nuclei for the formation of the Asian-Oceanian, the Latin American, the Pan-African, and the Pan-Arab neurological associations.

The structure of the proposed decentralized WFN

In van Bogaert's 1962 plan, the central governing body of the WFN was the group of WFN President and Officers, the Editor-in-Chief of the *Journal of the Neurological Sciences*, the Secretaries of Problem Commissions (still existing in 1962) and the Chairman of the Committee on Constitution.

The function of the Central Secretariat of the 1962 plan was to serve as the coordinating agency of three major regional associations, Greater European, Greater American, and Greater Asian-Oceania, collect Society dues and solicitation of funds, and act as the administrative and fiscal agent for organization of quadrennial international congresses. The regional associations would have their own secretariats and elect their own regional Vice Presidents and regional committees, all financed from regional sources.

The African continent was not included. This was in 1962. In 1960, the British Prime Minister Harold Macmillan had said 'The wind of change is blowing through this continent, and whether we like it or not, this growth of national consciousness is a political fact'. In the following years, former colonies became independent nations. For the WFN, however, the African continent apparently did not exist in 1960.

In 1957, Charles Poser became the WFN Medical Executive Officer. One of his duties was to undertake 'recruiting' trips in order to acquaint neurologists in other parts of the world with the general purposes of the WFN and enlist their support in getting their respective national neurological societies to join the federation (3).

The development of the AOAN differs considerably from that of the Greater American Region, although the regional associations were established almost simultaneously. The establishment of the Indian, Japanese, and Australian neurological societies became the key units in the formation of the AOAN, but it has to be borne in mind that the AOAN was formed only for the purpose of organizing the Tokyo Congress (4).

The candidates for the positions as Regional Directors are nominated by the Regional Associations of Neurology. It is the PAANS that selects the candidate for the African region, the AAN for the North American region, the Latin American Neurological Association for the Latin American region, the EFNS for the European region, the PAUNS for the East Mediterranean region, and the AOAN for the Asian-Oceania Region. The Council of Delegates formally appoints the Regional directors.

In 2005/2006, the Council of Delegates elected Jacques de Reuck (Belgium) as the European Regional Director, Thomas R. Swift (USA) the North American Regional Director, Mario Tolentino Dipp (Dominican Republic) the Latin American Regional Director, Bhim Sen Singhal (India) the Asian-Oceanian Regional Director, Ashraf Kurdi (Jordan) the Pan Arab Union and Gilbert Avode Doussou (Benin) the Pan-African Regional Director.

The positions of Regional Director may rotate with the function period for each candidate. Thus, in 2009 Ahmed Khalifa (Syria) succeeded Riadh Gouider (Tunisia), Robert Griggs (USA) succeeded Thomas Swift, Richard Hughes (UK) succeeded Jacques de Reuck, Alfred Njamnshi (Cameroon) succeeded Gilbert Avode Doussou, Ana Mercedes Robles de Hernandez succeeded Mario Tolentino Dipp, and Amado San Luis succeeded Bhim Sen Singhal.

The Asian Oceanian Association of Neurology (AOAN) (Greater Asian-Oceanian Association of Neurological Societies)

In 1959, Charles Poser visited Japan and India and challenged its neurologists to form an association that would promote and foster the advancement and exchange of neuro scientific information within the region (3–5).

Dr Shigeo Okinaka subsequently invited the region's neurologists to a planning meeting in Tokyo, Japan. This resulted in the birth of the AOAN on 26 June 1961.

The AOAN inaugural congress was held in Nippon Toshi Centre in Tokyo on 7–10 October 1962 under the leadership of Professor Okinaka. It was an outstanding success due to the organizational genius of the Japanese Committee, headed by Okinaka, the friendliness of the Japanese group, and the beauty of the country. The congress was sponsored by the WFN and the NINDB. Professor Okinaka, the founding Chairman of the Japanese Society of Neurology

REGIONAL NEUROLOGICAL ASSOCIATIONS | **153**

(JSN) and the first Japanese delegate to the WFN, also served as one of the WFN Regional Vice Presidents, representing Asia.

Since then, various countries have hosted the AOAN.

The 2nd congress was held in Melbourne, Australia, the 3rd took place in Bombay, India, the 4th in Bangkok, Thailand, followed by the 5th in Manila, Philippines, 6th in Taiwan, 7th in Bali, Indonesia, 8th in Tokyo, Japan, the 9th in Seoul, Korea, 10th in Manila, Philippines, 11th in Singapore and the 12th in New Delhi, India. In 2008, the WFN Council of Delegates was integrated in the Asian-Oceanian Congress that took place in New Delhi. Subsequent congresses are held every two years before and after each World Congress of Neurology. The present Chairman of the AOAN is Ching-Piao Tsai of Taiwan.

Current (2011) AOAN members are Australia and New Zealand, China, Hong Kong, India, Indonesia, Israel, Japan, Malaysia, Mongolia, Myanmar, Pakistan, Philippines, Saudi Arabia, Singapore, South Korea, Sri Lanka, Taiwan, Thailand, and Vietnam.

The Neurological Society of India

In the words of Man Mohan Mehndiratta:

> After India gained independence on August 15, 1947, it was not only a beginning of a new era for a young and developing India, it also marked the opening up of new horizons in the field of neurology. Till 1951 neurology was in a nascent stage and it was only after efforts of four young men, Dr Jacob Chandy, Dr B. Ramamurthi, Dr S.T. Narasimhan and Dr Baldev Singh, that the Neurological Society of India (NSI) was established.
>
> Jacob Chandy, B. Ramamurthi, S.T. Narasimhan and Baldev Singh conceptualized, created and constituted India's first neurological society. They brought all the disciplines associated with the science of neurology under one roof.
>
> Baldev Singh had trained in the USA and became based in New Delhi. Eddie Bharucha was the first neurologist in Bombay, and his wife Piroja a paediatrician. Noshir Wadia and Anil Desai were neurologists. Darab Dastur was a neuropathologist, and Jimmy Sidhwa a neuroradiologist. Most of the neurologists had trained in London, but Dastur had trained with Webb Haymaker in Washington (5).
>
> 30 members from all over the country attended the first meeting in Hyderabad, in 1952. Since its formation, the society has grown from strength to strength.
>
> Many milestones have been achieved, some deserve special mention.
>
> During the first meeting itself, *Indian Journal – Neurology*, which was later renamed *Neurology India*, came into existence. In 1963, NSI detached from the Association of Physicians of India. In 1972, the Sub-Committee for standardization of Postgraduate Education was formed.
>
> The year 1977 deserves special mention as this was the year when Neurophysiology / EEG sub-sections of the society were formed. It was decided to hold a Continuing Medical Education (CME) Programme, along with the annual conference with the intention of providing updates on selected topics and encouraging interdisciplinary interaction among trainees in the various branches of the Neurological Sciences. NSI

was probably the first medical professional society in the country to organize a formal CME programme section. Not only the neurological society grew at a national level, but recognition also came from international quarters. In 1989 the Society organized the World Congress of Neurology in New Delhi along with the 18th International Epilepsy Congress at New Delhi in October 1989. Eddie P. Bharucha was the Congress President, and Jagjit Chopra the Secretary- General.

In October 2008, the WFN organized its Council of Delegates during the joint 16th Annual Conference of the Indian Academy of Neurology and 12th Asian Oceania Congress of Neurology (AOCN) in New Delhi (Organizing Secretary of this joint conference was Professor Man Mohan Mehndiratta). A website for the society called www. neurosocietyindia.org was started in 1997. The journal *Neurology India* was placed online, the articles published and became available on the Internet from March 1997.

In 1992 a landmark development took place in the field of neurology when the Indian Academy of Neurology (IAN) came into existence. Since then many eminent personalities in the field of neurology have shared important posts and contributed significantly with their rich and vast experience. The IAN is affiliated to the WFN. It has taken great effort and time of these highly respected neurologists, what started as a group with a small number of members has now grown to a current strength of as many as 1200 members. Currently, close to 100 neurology trainees get qualified annually. IAN has a website www.ianindia.com and the journal *Annals of Indian Academy of Neurology* is available online with free access. Neurology in India is of an international standard and the majority of the specialty hospitals have state of the art technology.

To conclude from what started as a small activity, the Indian Academy of Neurology has now become an internationally acclaimed large family.

The Japanese Society of Neurology

This section was written with the assistance of Ryui Kaji, Shigeki Kuzuhara, and Jun Kimura.

The Japanese Society of Neurology had very close ties with the WFN from its inception.

There was already an established Japanese Society of Neurology when Charles Poser visited Japan as a special envoy from the WFN. Professor Kinnosuke Miura, a neurologist from the Department of Internal Medicine, and Professor Shuzo Kure, a psychiatrist from the Department of Psychiatry, the Imperial University of Tokyo, had established it in 1902.

Over the years, psychiatrists became predominant in the Society, and in 1935, the name was changed to the Japanese Society of Psychiatry and Neurology (JSPN). After the Second World War, Japanese neurologists wanted to create an organization independent of the JSPN. The Clinical Neurology Gathering was established in 1954, and held in conjunction with the Annual Meeting of the JSPN. Members overlapped between the two. The Medical Neurology Study Group was also established in 1956, and since then has been held every year in conjunction with the Annual Meeting of the Japanese Society of Internal Medicine, with membership overlapping.

At the 5th Annual Meeting of the Medical Neurology Study Group in 1959, a renewed Japanese Society of Neurology was established with Charles M. Poser representing the WFN. The society was recognized as the Japanese branch of the WFN immediately following the first renewed JSN Annual Meeting in 1960.

In 1981, Professor Tadao Tsubaki, the second Chairman of the JSN, and Professor Yasuo Toyokura, then the Japanese delegate to the WFN, successfully invited the World Congress of Neurology to Japan. The 12th World Congress of Neurology—the 7th International Congress of Neurology took place in Kyoto in 1981. Shibanosuke Katsuki was the President, and Tadao Tsubaki Secretary-General. The Kyoto Congress preceded the International Congress of EEG and Clinical Neurophysiology (X-ICECN), a meeting organized by the IFCN. Success of this joint venture prompted another similar arrangement in Vancouver between XV-WCN and XIII-ICECN in 1993 (6).

When the WFN found it difficult to support the printing of *World Neurology*, Lord Walton, who was the President of the WFN, asked the delegates to look for external sponsorships. In response, Dr Eijiro Satoyoshi arranged for the Eisai Pharmaceutical Company in Japan to support publication for several years. Much later, during Kimura's tenure as WFN President, the WFN again faced a shortage of funds to cover the cost of the journal in view of expanding allocation of available resources for various global educational activities. After retiring from Toho University, Dr Satoyoshi became the head of the Japan Foundation for Neuroscience and Mental Health, which served as a vehicle to support fundraising for various neurological meetings. Having organized a number of national and international conferences with considerable fiscal success, Kimura had deposited the surplus with this foundation for future academic use in accordance with governmental regulation in Japan. Dr Satoyoshi and Kimura hoped to donate part of this sum to the WFN cause. After a series of negotiations, they were able to divert US$50,000 per year for five years from 2003 through 2007. Thanks to this initiative, the WFN could maintain the publication of *World Neurology* until the journal became self-supporting using income from advertising (6).

The Australian Association of Neurologists

The Australian Association of Neurologists was founded in Melbourne in 1950 (7). Leonard Bell Cox (1894–1976) was the first President. Edward Graeme Robertson (1903–1975), who worked at Queen Square in London 1930–1934, and became one of the leading authorities on pneumoencephalography, was also one of the founders. Cox and Graeme Robertson represented Melbourne. New Zealand members were also welcome, and the Australian and New Zealand Association of Neurologists merged in 2006.

Graeme Robertson was a very active member of the WFN from the beginning, and he was Regional Vice President during van Bogaert's Presidency. Australia was a founding member of the Asian-Oceanian Association of Neurology, and hosted the second AOAN congress in Melbourne in 1967. William Carroll was elected Trustee in London in 2001. The 18th World Congress of Neurology took place in Sydney in 2005. William Carroll (Perth) was the President, Geoffrey Donnan (Melbourne) Secretary-General, and Sam Berkovic (Melbourne) Chairman of the Scientific Programme Committee.

The WFN Asia Initiative

In his 2010 inauguration speech, WFN President Vladimir Hachinski conveyed a clear message:

> Asia has more than 60% of the global population, yet in some areas, the education of neurology to young neurologists does not keep up with the patients' needs of neurological care. For this reason, it is essential for WFN to help vitalize the education to promote activity on this region among others.
>
> Since I was appointed as the head of the Asia Initiative, I have been trying to promote the educational activities in neurology with the aid of many friends inside and outside Asia. It is for this reason that I invite you to attend the Asian-Oceanian Congress of Neurology (AOCN) 2012 meeting in Melbourne, Australia, June 4–8.
>
> Prof. Matthew Kiernan of Australia, the AOCN programme chair, and Prof. Ching Piao Tsai of Taiwan, the President of the Asian-Oceanian Association of Neurology (AOAN), are trying their best to plan an attractive programme with speakers from all over the world for AOCN and other educational courses, and to find as many sponsors as possible to improve the financial status of the meeting. Prof. Tsai and his colleagues have decided to hold the AOCN every two years instead of every four years, and if the congress is a success, future meetings could attract more and more people over the years, and might be held every year. A successful meeting will mean that Asian and Oceanian societies are now getting closer to becoming a unified neurology organization.
>
> I have talked with Prof. Tsai and his colleagues, and it is clear that we share a dream of having an annual meeting in the future that is comparable with the European Federation of Neurological Societies congress in Europe, or the American Academy of Neurology meeting in North America.
>
> We met last November at the World Congress of Neurology in Marrakesh, Morocco, and had an Asia Initiative meeting. A total of 17 people from inside and outside the region attended the meeting and had many productive discussions. We reached three major points to pursue in our future activities.
>
> First, it is important for associations to hold meetings in collaboration with one another. It is strategically important to use existing frameworks, including AOCN. We could ask the ASEAN (Association of Southeast Asian Nations) Neurological Association, which is headed by Prof. C. Tan of Indonesia (an informal get-together of those from Korea, Taiwan, China, Hong Kong, and Japan) to synchronize meetings, so that a large attendance can be expected. Joint meetings between any of these two organizations are now being planned for the 2014 AOCN meeting in Hong Kong.

Second, it is essential to work with other international organizations, such as the Movement Disorder Society or the International Federation of Clinical Neurophysiology. Both of these organizations have agreed to have a satellite basic movement disorder course or a basic EMG hands-on course at the AOCN 2012 meeting.

Third, we will ask groups of young neurologists to join these activities through the Internet. Dr Tissa Wijeratne of Australia, who also represents Sri Lankan neurologists, proposed this promising idea. He is now forming the Asia Pacific Association of Young Neurologists and Trainees.

We need your help for this dream, which also embodies that of WFN itself. Please come and join AOCN 2012 for a wide variety of educational opportunities at a reasonable cost for travel, accommodation, and registration.

Ryuji Kaji (8)

The Pan American Association of Neurology

Van Bogaert called it the 'Greater American' section of the WFN: Greater American Association of Neurological Societies (North, South, Central American and Mexico).

During the preparations for the International Congress of Neurological Sciences in Brussels in 1957, letters of invitation were sent to national neurological societies throughout the world. The letters informed them that there would be an organizational meeting during this congress and invited them to have a delegate at the meeting. Among the 38 delegates who came to the meeting were representatives from 29 national societies, six of them from Latin American countries (Argentina, Brazil, Chile, Cuba, Peru, Uruguay). For comparison, there were two neurologists from the USA, one from South Africa and two from Asia (Iran and India) (Chapter 2).

At the Brussels meeting, and even more so after the Federation had been established, van Bogaert and the WFN administration had pointed out the importance of having regional neurology organizations. The Pan American and the Asian-Oceanian regions were obvious candidates. Charles Poser had already visited India and Japan on behalf of the Antwerp office.

Why was Latin America so well represented at the foundation of the WFN? One reason is that neurology in Latin America was already well developed. There were advanced neuroscience centres in Argentina, Brazil, Chile, Peru, and Uruguay. José Pereyra-Käfer, who attended the Brussels conference, was a neurology professor at the University of Buenos Aires and had founded the Sociedad Neurológica Argentina in 1952.

The first neurological institute in Latin America, the Instituto de Neurologia de Montevideo in Uruguay, was founded as early as 1927, and Roman Arana-Iñiguez, who also attended the Brussels congress, was the Institute's third director. Oscar Trelles Montes from Lima, Peru, had trained with Jean Lhermitte in

Paris from 1930 to 1935. He was a professor of neuropathology in Lima, and was one of the founders of Sociedad Peruana de Psiqiatria, Neurologia y Neurochirurgia, which consisted mainly of neurologists. Deolindo Couto, who also attended the Brussels congress, was the first president of the Academia Brasileira de Neurologia. Alfonso Asenjo from Chile, who had trained with Walter Dandy (1886–1946) in the USA and with Wilhelm Tönnis (1898–1978) in Germany, became the director of the Institute of Neurosurgery and Brain Research in Santiago, Chile in 1953, and was new in the position when he left for Brussels. He remained, however, the Director for 34 years (9,10).

Venezuela, Colombia, Bolivia, and Ecuador were not represented at the WFN foundation meeting, but all four countries also had well-trained neurologists and neurological/neurosurgical departments. Manuel Guevara of Mexico City became professor of neurology in Mexico in 1929. Francisco Rubio Donnadieu, who had trained at the National Hospital in London, consolidated neurology in Mexico. He became the president of the Consejo Mexicano de Neurología, which became the largest training centre for specialists in Latin America (10).

The First Pan American Congress of Neurology (Lima, Peru, October 20–25, 1963)

In Rome in 1961, Professor Alfonso Asenjo Gómez (Santiago de Chile) and Dr Gustavo Poch (Buenos Aires) met to discuss the feasibility of organizing Pan American Congresses of Neurology under the auspices of the WFN, and to be held at four-yearly intervals between the international congresses of neurology. A few days later, they met with Professor Oscar Trelles in Lima, Peru. Trelles, who was enthusiastic about the idea, became the Prime Minister of Peru and thereafter was appointed Peruvian Ambassador to France.

A few months later, at the meeting of the WFN Problem Commission on Tropical Neurology in Buenos Aires, a Pan American Organization Committee was formed. The Committee Representatives from Argentina, Brazil, Uruguay, Chile, Peru, and the USA convened and discussed the plans. Professor Trelles was elected President, with the WFN President, Dr Ludo van Bogaert, *ex officio* member of the Committee. The Committee formulated tentative plans including the scientific programme, and it was decided that the Congress should take place in Lima, Peru, in the latter part of October 1963. The National Institute of Neurological Diseases and Blindness made a substantial grant of US$31,000 to help promulgate the congress and publish the transactions. Additional financial support was received from the Peruvian Government, local societies, and the WFN.

The Congress was inaugurated in the Salón de las Américas, Palacio Municipal, Lima, in the presence of the Constitutional President of the Republic of Peru, Arquitecto Fernando Belaúnde Terry. It was held under the auspices of the Peruvian Government, the WFN, and the National Institute of Neurological Diseases and Blindness.

President Oscar Trelles gave the Inaugural Address, followed by the WFN Vice President, Professor Raymond Garcin (Paris). The President, His Excellency Belaúnde Terry, gave the final speech and welcomed the members of the Congress for a buffet reception as guests of President Belaúnde in the historic and palatial setting of the Governor's Palace.

Congress participation

The Executive Committee consisted of the national WFN delegates from the neurological societies of the various countries of the Americas. There were 500 registrations.

Unfortunately, the WFN President, Ludo van Bogaert, was unable to attend the Congress, but he inspired the group with a telegram of good wishes and welcomed the installation of the American Continental Group of the WFN at the occasion of the First Pan American Congress of Neurology. Fortunately, the WFN Vice President Professor Raymond Garcin (France) could attend and participated in the sessions. The WFN Secretary-Treasurer General, Percival Bailey (Chicago), served as Honorary President. Professors Deolindo Couto (Rio de Janeiro), Hugo Lea-Plaza (Santiago), H. Houston Merritt (New York), Wilder Penfield (Princeton), A.L. Sahs (Iowa City), and Marcelino Sepich (Buenos Aires) were also Honorary Presidents. Armand Lowenthal (Antwerp, Belgium) came as a special WFN emissary.

Scientific Sessions: The scientific sessions lasted for 5 days and were held in the conference rooms of Lima's Gran Hotel Bolivár. The major topics were:

1 clinical and biological aspects of neuromuscular disease

2 neurological manifestations of internal, toxic, and dysmetabolic diseases

3 special conferences, related to alternations of consciousness (Lhermitte, Paris), copper metabolism (Lowenthal), hypertensive encephalopathy and cerebral oedema (Garcin, Paris, and Gilliatt, London), and neurological education (Gozzano, Rome).

WFN executive sessions

At the request of the WFN President, Ludo van Bogaert, Professor Trelles called two WFN Executive Meetings to select the venue for the next Pan American Congress of Neurology (1967), and to discuss the WFN decentralization plan. By unanimous vote, it was decided that the Second Pan American Congress of Neurology should take place in San Juan (Puerto Rico) under the Presidency of Luis P. Sánchez-Longo. This came as a suggestion from Professor Trelles on the grounds that the 9th International Congress of Neurology (1969) would take place in the USA, which would result in an uneven distribution between the northern and southern hemispheres. He believed that these congresses should alternate between English and Spanish speaking countries (11).

In the discussion about an equitable distribution of the congresses between North and Latin America, the area of Panama was arbitrarily selected as a line of demarcation between the two hemispheres; the societies of all countries south of Panama should be regarded as the southern group, while societies in areas north of Panama should be regarded as the northern group.

In the name of Puerto Rico and the Puerto Rican Academy of Neurology, Professor Sánchez-Longo thanked the delegates for the honour of designating the Commonwealth of Puerto Rico as the site for the Second Pan-American Congress of Neurology.

The First Pan-American Congress of Neurology was a success, because of the leadership of President Oscar Trelles and his local Executive Committee, and also because of the high quality of the presentations given. As in all activities of the WFN during the early part of its existence, assistance and financial support from the National Institute of Neurological Diseases and Blindness was a critical element in the formative period of the federation.

The second Pan-American Congress of Neurology was held in San Juan de Puerto Rico in 1967 with Luis P. Sanchez Longo as President, the third in Sao Paulo, Brazil, 1971, and the fourth in Mexico City 1975 with Francisco Rubio Donnadieu as President. The President of Mexico Luis Echeverra inaugurated the congress with the attendance of 1200 participants, including more than 500 Americans and Canadians and 300 from Central America and South America. Subsequent Pan American Congresses have been held in Caracas (1979), Buenos Aires (1983), San Juan, Puerto Rico (1987), Montevideo (1991), Guatemala City (1995), Cartagena, Columbia (1999), Santiago, Chile (2003), and Santo Domingo, Dominican Republic, (2007).

The Pan African Association of Neurological Sciences (PAANS)

One African neurologist attended the inauguration ceremony of the WFN in Brussels in 1957. He was Sam Berman, head of the neuropsychiatry department at Groote Sehum Hospital in Cape Town. Berman had received his full neurology training in London, UK. He died in 1963. The apartheid system meant that there was a split in the patient population, and there was no contact with the health systems in other English-speaking countries in Africa.

The Pan African Association of Neurological Sciences (PAANS) was founded in Nairobi, Kenya, in 1972. Its main function is the advancement of neurological sciences and the promotion of friendship and exchange amongst practitioners of and people interested in neurological sciences in Africa in particular and in the world at large (12).

In 1972, Professor Renato Ruberti of Kenya organized a symposium in Nairobi on tumours of the nervous system in different parts of Africa. At the end of that meeting, PAANS was formed 'to promote the neurosciences in the whole of Africa – from Cairo in the north to Cape Town in the south and from Somalia and the Horn of Africa in the east to Senegambia in the west. Scientific meetings of the Association would be held once in two years, with the venue alternating between Anglophone and Francophone countries' (12). Osman Sorour of Cairo was elected President, and Renato Ruberti of Nairobi Secretary-General.

The first PAANS Congress was held in Cairo in 1973. Membership of PAANS is open to specialists in neurology, neurosurgery, neuropsychiatry, neuroradiology, neuropathology, neuropharmacology, neurobiochemistry, neuroanatomy, neurophysiology or in one of the neurosciences acceptable to the Executive Council.

When PAANS applied for membership of the WFN, the WFN decided that, being a continental body, it would not have voting rights. The World Federation of Neurosurgical Societies (WFNS) took the opposite decision. There is no doubt that the contacts between PAANS and the WFNS have been stronger than they have been between PAANS and the WFN. PAANS has characterized the relationship with the WFNS as 'harmonious and productive', and the WFNS was involved early in plans for organizing training courses in neurosurgery in Africa. The President of the WFN, Richard Masland, invited every African country with five or more neurologists (including neurosurgeons) to apply for WFN membership and have a WFN delegate with the right to vote. Countries with fewer than five neurologists would be represented by PAANS.

PAANS has two sections, a neurology section, and a neurosurgery section, and delegates to the WFN and WFNS are eligible as delegates according to background. For practical reasons, when the PAANS President is a neurosurgeon, the Vice President usually takes on the functions related to neurology and vice versa.

Individual African countries with neurologists were invited to apply for membership, and the Nigerian Society of Neurological Sciences, formed in 1966, was already a WFN member at the birth of PAANS. Algeria and Libya now became WFN members. There was no PAUNS society at that time.

The Second PAANS congress was held in Dakar, Senegal, in 1975. Henri Collomb and Michel Dumas chaired the meeting, where Morocco and Tunisia became new member societies, and Michel Dumas was elected new PAANS President.

At the Third PAANS Congress, in Lagos, Nigeria in 1977, Olufemi Dada was elected new PAANS President. At the Lagos meeting, the neurological societies of Nigeria, Senegal, Kenya, Egypt, Tunisia, Morocco, and South Africa were registered PAANS members in addition to the neurosurgical society of South Africa.

The Fourth PAANS Congress took place in Algiers, Algeria, in 1979, and M. Abada of Algeria was elected President. Madagascar became the 20th member country joining PAANS. Nairobi, Kenya, was the venue of the 5th PAANS Congress, in 1981. Somalia and Rwanda now joined the organization, and Renato Ruberti was elected PAANS President. The 6th PAANS Congress took place in Tunisia in 1983. Mongi Ben-Hamida was elected new President. This was the first PAANS conference with simultaneous English–French and French–English translations.

Tanzania became a new PAANS member in 1983. There was no PAANS Congress in Zimbabwe in 1985, as had been planned, and the 7th PAANS Congress was organized in Abidjan, Ivory Coast. Christian Giordano of the Ivory Coast became the next PAANS President. Subsequent PAANS congresses were held in Accra (Ghana) in 1988, where Sierra Leone and Benin were admitted, and in Harare, Zimbabwe, in 1990. The 10th PAANS Congress was held in Marrakesh, Morocco, in 1992, under the high patronage of His Majesty King Hassan II. Registration took place in Casablanca, and was then moved to Marrakesh. Professor Najat Boukhrissi was elected President, the first time PAANS was privileged to have a lady as President. Congo and Niger were admitted new member societies.

The 11th PAANS Congress took place in Addis Ababa, Ethiopia, in 1994, when Redda Tekle Haimanot was elected President, the 12th in Durban, South Africa, in 1996, with Pierre Bill as President, the 13th in Dakar, Senegal, 1998, with Ibrahima P. Ndiaye as President, the 14th in Blantyre, Malawi, in 2000, where Adelola Adeloye was elected President, the 15th in Cairo, Egypt in 2002 with Sayed El-Gindi as President, the 16th in 2004 in Cotonou, Benin, the 17th in Lagos, Nigeria in 2006, and the 18th in Yaoundé, Cameroon in 2008. The 19th PAANS Congress was planned in Tripoli, Libya, but cancelled because of the disturbing political developments.

The Africa Initiative

The Africa Initiative was launched at the Africa meeting in London in December 2006. It is a collective term used for describing various WFN activities related to the development of neurology in sub-Saharan Africa, such as training of new neurologists, establishing educational programmes in neurology, supporting new national neurological associations, assistance in fund-raising for neurology in this part of the world, travelling fellowships, support of public health activities in sub-Saharan Africa, and collaboration with WHO, EFNS, and IBRO.

The basic task is the training of neurologists on the African continent. For French-speaking African countries, training of neurologists will mainly be in Senegal, Morocco, and Tunisia, while training of neurologists from the English-speaking countries can take place in Egypt and South Africa.

A main problem is the lack of medical schools with a neurology programme in sub-Saharan Africa. This is the main reason why there are so few neurologists trained in their home country. Apparently, the lack of basic neuroscience courses at the medical schools serves as an impediment to effective graduation of neurologists. This is one of the reasons for the agreements made with medical schools in Egypt, Morocco, and Tunisia. During the practical organization of the project, the WFN has had a close collaboration with the PAUNS. From the very beginning, the PAUNS countries have been strongly involved and have been very helpful. Thanks to their assistance, we have obtained funds for future neurology training. The next link will be the selection of candidates with proper prioritization, and funding of the training expenses. Public health challenges are important in sub-Saharan neurology, and national health authorities will have to be involved as there are already a few individual national neurological societies and the IBRO.

The situation for neurologists in Africa was discussed by the WFN membership committee and at the Council of Delegates in Stockholm in 2012. The number of specialists in neurology is clearly lower in Africa than in the other WHO regions. The median number of neurologists per 100 000 population is extremely low in Africa, 0.03 versus 0.07 in South-East Asia, 0.32 in the Eastern Mediterranean, 0.77 in the Western Pacific, 0.89 in the Americas, and 4.84 in Europe. The WHO has thus demonstrated a lack of trained neurologists in Africa.

The Africa Initiative Committee met during the Congress, and there was agreement to increase the training of neurologists in Africa, and especially in Ghana and Tanzania, and establish a closer contact with the relevant medical schools. Neither country had a neurological society nor was a member of the

WFN. Both collaborated with ILAE, had major medical schools and facilities, and were capable of supporting training programmes.

The Pan Arab Union of Neurological Societies (PAUNS)

Ahmed Khalifa writes that:

The Pan Arab region spans across the Middle East, Near East and North Africa with many shared interests in both continents. The estimated total population of the Arab world was around 318 million in 2005, which numerically is roughly equivalent to the North American Population. The region comprises 23 countries and the total number of neurologists varies from nil e.g. Djibouti and Somalia to 1:40,000 in Lebanon.

The idea of a Pan Arab union of neurosciences arose in 1973 during the World Congress of Neurology held in Barcelona, when some representatives from Arab countries attending that congress met and discussed the idea, but it was not until 1975 that PAUNS became a reality.

That year, the Egyptian Society of Neurology, Psychiatry and Neurosurgery held the first Pan Arab meeting of Neurosciences, in Cairo, and there was agreement to create the new organization, called the Pan Arab Union of Neurosciences. Professor Ahmed El-Benhawy, Ain Shams, Cairo was nominated as the first president in May 1975.

Since 1975, twelve Pan Arab Congresses have been held in different parts of the Arab World, all under the auspices of the WFN. The last one took place in Damascus, Syria, in May 2010.

In 1984, Arab psychiatrists formed a Pan Arab Psychiatric Association. The Pan Arab Neuroradiological Society was formed in 1994. In 1995 the Arab Neurosurgical Society was founded, followed by the Pan Arab Pediatric Neurology Society. After the PAUNS meeting in Riyadh in 1997, the name of the Pan Arab Union of Neurosciences was changed to the Pan Arab Union of Neurological Societies, keeping the same abbreviation: PAUNS.

An important achievement is the establishment of a PAUNS symposium at each World Congress of Neurology, starting from London, 2001(chaired by Saleh El-Deeb), then Sydney, 2005 (chaired by Anwar Etribi), and Bangkok, 2009 (chaired by Ryadh Gouider). Ahmed Khalifa, chaired the symposium in Marrakesh, Morocco, in 2010.

The official Journal of PAUNS is *Neurosciences* produced by the Saudi Society of Neurology.

Since its establishment in 1975, PAUNS has been chaired by the following Presidents: Ahmed El-Banhawy, Egypt, Ashraf El-Kurdi, Jordan, El-Monji Ben Hamida, Tunisia, Emad Fadli, Egypt, Saleh El-Deeb, Saudi Arabia, Anwar Etribi, Egypt, Saher Hashem, Egypt, Riadh Gouider, Tunisia, and Ahmed Khalifa, Syria.

The European Federation of Neurological Societies (EFNS)

The Greater European Association of Neurological Societies (Britain, Europe, and USSR) was slow to develop. Neurology was relatively well organized, and the WFN was established and formed in Europe. Europe was, however, still split, and most western European countries had a much closer contact with the USA than with eastern Europe. Several European neurologists are and were then already members of the AAN and attended their annual meetings. Some former Communist countries of East Europe, especially Czechoslovakia, Hungary and Poland had a closer contact with the west than for example Romania and Ukraine. This has probably historic roots related to existing pre-Soviet contacts and the training of neurologists before 1914.

In 1960, the WFN had accepted the German Democratic Republic (GDR) and the GDR-Section of the WFN was founded in East Berlin the same year. The WFN President, Ludo van Bogaert, who was from Belgium, was invited, and the organizers even bought a Belgian flag for the occasion. The West German neurologists were, however, unaware that the WFN had already accepted the GDR in 1960. This may have delayed the diplomatic process whereby the WFN accepted a separate GDR section.

Many European neurologists now hoped for a better integration of neurosciences in Europe. In 1986, Professor Miecyslaw Wender of Poznan, Poland, proposed a unified European Neurological Society. In 1989, Professor Daniel Bartko of Bratislava, and Franz Gerstenbrand of Innsbruck organized the first Pan-European congress for neurology in Prague in 1989. There were near 1500 attendees. Gerstenbrand, Bartko, and Alessandro Agnoli, Rome, first proposed the formation of the Pan-European Society of Neurology.

In an attempt to merge the two, Professor Franz Gerstenbrand (Innsbruck, Austria) took the initiative to form a European Federation of Neurological Societies (EFNS), which had its first congress in Vienna in December 1991 and it was also the Second Pan-European Congress as well as the 1st EFNS Congress. Its location was the Wiener Hofburg, and Franz Gerstenbrand was the President.

The main principles for the content of the programme and the invitation of speakers were to select highly qualified speakers for excellent topics. The speakers were invited to Vienna from all over Europe, as well as from the USA. In his welcoming speech, Professor Gerstenbrand announced the foundation of a European Federation of Neurological Societies, and Council of Delegates consisting of representatives of each national European society. The next EFNS congresses were held in Berlin (1993), Poznan (1994), Marseilles (1995), Rome (1996), Prague (1997), Seville (1998), Lisbon (1999), Copenhagen (2000), Vienna (2002), Helsinki (2003), Paris (2004), Athens (2005), Glasgow (2006), Brussels (2007), Madrid (2008), Florence (2009), Geneva (2010), Budapest (2011), and Stockholm (2012).

The structure and constitution of the EFNS was accomplished by the loyal and solid teamwork of Professor Gerstenbrand, Dr Frederieke Tschabitscher, and the Management Committee and Professor Jes Olesen, the second President of the EFNS. During Professor Olesen's presidency, several new committees were set up. They established contact with the European Union, of which most EFNS countries are members.

The EFNS has a strong relationship with the WFN, regulated in the constitution. The collaboration with the WFN is well organized, and there will be no EFNS congress in years when the World Congress takes place in a European country (2001, 2013).

The European Neurological Society (ENS)

At the same time, a group of young, vigorous neurologists from France and the UK, including Gerard Said of Paris, P.K. Thomas, and Anita Harding from London, decided to launch an organization which would function as the ENS for individual members, owing no specific allegiance to the national societies. The ENS congresses are of a high quality. However, there are currently (2012) plans for merging the ENS and EFNS during the next four to five years. The new organization will probably be named the European Academy of Neurology.

References

1 **Wadia N.** *Neurological Practice: An Indian Perspective*. Elsevier 2005.

2 **Cohen MM.** Presidents of the American Academy of Neurology. In MM Cohen Ed. *The American Academy of Neurology: The first 50 years, 1949–1998*. American Academy of Neurology.

3 **Poser CM.** The World Federation of Neurology: the formative period 1955–1961. Personal recollections. *J Neurol Sci* 1993; **120**: 218–27.

4 **Bailey P.** Meeting of the WFN Executive Committee (El Escorial, Madrid, Spain, May 8–9, 1964). *J Neurol Sci* 1965; **2**: 293–96.

5 **Poser CM.** Neurology in the developing world. *Brain* 2006; **129**:1624–9.

6 **Kimura J.** Personal Communication 2010.

7 **Foley PB, Storey C.** History of neurology in Australia and New Zealand. In S. Finger, F. Boller, K.L. Tyler Eds. *Handbook of Clinical Neurology*, Vol. 95. *History of Neurology*. 2010, pp. 781–800.

8 **Allegri R.** The pioneers of clinical neurology in South America. *J Neurol Sci* 2008; **271**: 29–33.

9 **Allegri R.** Clinical neurology in Latin America. In S. Finger, F. Boller, K.L. Tyler Eds. *Handbook of Clinical Neurology*, Vol. 95. *History of Neurology*. 2010, pp. 801–14.

10 **Bailey P.** Report on the first Pan American Congress of Neurology (Lima, Peru, October 20–25, 1963). *J Neurol Sci* 1965 **2**: 203–12.

11 **Adeloye A, Ruberti R.** *The Pan African Association of Neurological Sciences (PAANS). The First Thirty Years*. BookBuilders, Ibadan 2008.

Chapter 7

The World Federation of Neurology and the World Health Organization

Representatives of 50 countries met in San Francisco in 1945, and one important topic was the need for a global health organization. The World Health Organization—WHO—was established. It became the directing and coordinating authority for health within the United Nations. The WHO constitution came into force on 7 April 1948—which we celebrate as World Health Day.

The WHO is the directing and coordinating authority for health within the United Nations. More than 8000 people from more than 150 countries work for the Organization in 147 country offices, six regional offices, and at the headquarters in Geneva, Switzerland, and correspond closely with national health authorities.

The WFN regions

The WHO structure is based upon political, social, economic, and other factors still relevant in 2011. The member countries are grouped in six WHO regions: the African region, the region of the Americas, the South-East Asia region, the European region, the Eastern Mediterranean region, and the Western Pacific region (1).

The WFN regions are crucial in the discussions about the structure of the WFN. Regional Vice Presidents have been elected since 1965, but until 2001, the Council of Delegates elected them, without their function being defined. Nor did they represent the respective regional neurological associations— except for their function as the editorial board of *World Neurology*.

When Johan Aarli was elected First Vice President in 2001, he initiated a comprehensive discussion on the relationship between the WFN central administration and the Regional Vice Presidents. By 2003, the Trustees had arrived at a new definition for the Regional Vice Presidents, which was approved by the WFN Council of Delegates in Sydney. The discussions at the Council of Delegates 2003 made it clear that the Regional Vice Presidents would have a stronger basis when representing a regional neurological association. No changes were introduced, as the current Regional Vice Presidents were then mid-way through their terms of office. The WFN did, however, prefer the term Regional Director and not Regional Vice President. This also involved definitions of the regions, and the WFN decided to follow the structure of the WHO.

The WFN has a close collaboration with the WHO, which is responsible for providing leadership on global health matters and shaping the health research agenda. It is important for the WFN with its geographical and regional programmes to operate within the WHO geography.

Each WHO region has a regional office, in Brazzaville, Congo, for the African region, in New Delhi, India, for the South-East Asian region, in Washington, DC, for the American region, in Copenhagen, Denmark, for the European region, in Cairo, Egypt, for the Eastern Mediterranean region, and in Manila, Philippines, for the Western Pacific region.

The WFN is among 182 different non-governmental organizations (NGOs) in official relations with the WHO, and it has adopted a regional system that in principle is based upon the WHO structure. There are two main differences. The WFN has found it practical to have two WFN regions for the Americas: the Latin American and the North American region. The WFN Asian-Oceania region is based upon two WHO regions, South-East Asia and the Western Pacific region, while the WFN AO has decided to remain in one region.

The WHO structure was drawn up in 1948, and is based upon political, social, economic, and other factors that are still relevant in 2011. The WHO African region comprises 46 Member States: Algeria, Angola, Benin, Botswana, Burkina Faso, Burundi, Cameroon, Cape Verde, Central African Republic, Chad, Comoros, Congo, Cote d'Ivoire, Democratic Republic of Congo, Equatorial Guinea, Eritrea, Ethiopia, Gabon, Gambia, Ghana, Guinea, Guinea-Bissau, Kenya, Lesotho, Liberia, Madagascar, Malawi, Mali, Mauritania, Mauritius, Mozambique, Namibia, Niger, Nigeria, Rwanda, São Tomé & Príncipe, Senegal, Seychelles, Sierra Leone, South Africa, Swaziland, Tanzania, Togo, Uganda, Zambia, and Zimbabwe.

According to the WHO structure, Algeria is a part of the WHO African and not of the Eastern Mediterranean region, while Morocco, Tunisia, Libya, Egypt, Eritrea, Sudan, and Somalia are outside the WHO African region.

The WHO Eastern Mediterranean region comprises the following national states: Afghanistan, Bahrain, Djibouti, Egypt, Arab Republic of Iran, Iraq, Jordan, Kuwait, Lebanon, Libya, Morocco, Oman, Pakistan, Palestine, Qatar, Saudi Arabia, Somalia, Sudan, Syrian Arab Republic, Tunisia, United Arab Emirates, and Yemen.

The WHO South-East Asia region comprises 11 national states: Bangladesh, Bhutan, Democratic People's Republic of Korea, India, Indonesia, Maldives,

THE WORLD FEDERATION OF NEUROLOGY AND THE WORLD HEALTH ORGANIZATION | **169**

Myanmar, Nepal, Sri Lanka, Thailand, and Timor Leste. The WHO Western Pacific region is huge, with approximately 1.6 billion inhabitants and nearly one-third of the world's population: American Samoa, Australia, Brunei, Cambodia, China, Cook Islands, Fiji, French Polynesia, Guam, Hong Kong, Japan, Kiribati, Lao People's Democratic Republic, Macao, Malaysia, Micronesia, Mongolia, Nauru, New Caledonia, New Zealand, Niue, Northern Mariana Islands, Palau, Papua, Philippines, Pitcairn Island, Republic of Korea, Samoa, Singapore, Solomon Island, Tokelau, Tonga, Tuvalo, Vanuatu, Viet Nam, Wallis & Fortuna.

The WHO region of the Americas comprises Anguilla, Antigua and Barbuda, Argentina, Aruba, Bahamas, Barbados, Belize, Bermuda, Bolivia, Brazil, British Virgin Islands, Canada, Cayman Islands, Chile, Columbia, Costa Rica, Cuba, Dominica, Dominican Republic, El Salvador, Ecuador, US/Mexico Border, French Guiana, Grenada, Guadeloupe, Guatemala, Guyana, Haiti, Honduras, Jamaica, Martinique, Mexico, Montserrat, Netherlands Antilles, Nicaragua, Panama, Paraguay, Peru, Puerto Rico, Saint Kitts and Nevis, Saint Lucia, Saint Vincent and the Grenadines, Suriname, Trinidad & Tobago, Turks & Caicos Islands, Uruguay, Venezuela, USA.

The WHO European region comprises Albania, Andorra, Armenia, Austria, Azerbaijan, Belarus, Belgium, Bosnia and Herzegovina, Bulgaria, Croatia, Cyprus, Czech Republic, Denmark, Estonia, Finland, France, Georgia, Germany, Hungary, Iceland, Ireland, Israel, Italy, Kazakhstan, Kyrgyzstan, Latvia, Lithuania, Luxembourg, Malta, Monaco, Montenegro, Netherlands, Norway, Poland, Portugal, Republic of Moldova, Romania, Russian Federation, San Marino, Serbia, Slovakia, Slovenia, Spain, Sweden, Switzerland, Tajikistan, the former Yugoslav Republic of Macedonia, Turkey, Turkmenistan, Ukraine, United Kingdom of Great Britain and Northern Ireland, Uzbekistan.

'There is no health without mental health'

The WHO is not structured according to clinical specialties in medicine, and its structure has developed over the years. The WHO is the lead international agency responsible for health and is increasingly recognizing with the importance of mental health. The WFN is mainly concerned with performance in neurology, while the WHO's main responsibility is for public health.

Unfortunately, the term 'mental health' has been used euphemistically to describe treatment and support service for people with mental illness in general. This usage has added to the confusion about the concept of mental health as well as that of mental illness and led to a misconception that the WHO Division of Mental Health is an organization related specifically to psychiatry (2). To many neurologists, the term 'brain health' is a biologically more adequate term than 'mental health'. The structural units of the WHO are, however, not based upon clinical specialties. To decision-makers in governments at local and national levels, the term 'mental health' may offer political and practical advantages. The Division of Mental Health is organized as an integral part of Noncommunicable Diseases and Mental Health, which focuses upon mental health, substance abuse, and neurological disorders.

The WHO neuroscience meetings

The relationship between the WFN and the WHO has not always been uncomplicated. When Richard Masland took over as WFN President in 1981, one of his main challenges was to improve the relationship with the WHO. One challenge was the definition of 'mental health'. It was in Walton's presidency (1989–1997) that the head of the Division of Mental Health of the WHO, Norman Sartorius, invited the leaders of NGOs in neurosciences for an annual meeting near the end of the year. Walton's successor, James Toole, realized that such contact meetings with the WHO in Geneva could serve as a door opener for future contacts and subsequent collaboration between the WFN and the WHO. The leadership of the WHO Division of Mental Health and representatives has from the beginning attended the WHO neuroscience meetings from the neuroscience NGOs in official relationship with the WHO.

The *Global Burden of Disease* report drew the attention of the international health community to the fact that the burden of mental and neurological disorders has been seriously underestimated by traditional epidemiological methods. Jun Kimura, while WFN President, invited Aarli, first as the Chair of the WFN Public Relations Committee, then as the WFN First Vice President, to serve as the Liaison Officer between the WFN and the WHO. Following the Global Initiative on Neurology and Public Health, the Project Atlas was launched, with the object of collecting, compiling, and disseminating relevant information on health-care resources in countries. The work included 109 countries spanning all WHO regions and covering over 90% of the world population.

The *Neurology Atlas* showed that the available resources for neurological disorders in the world are insufficient when set against the known significant burden associated with these disorders. In addition, there are large inequities across regions and income groups in different countries, with low-income countries having extremely meagre resources (3).

The *Neurology Atlas* was followed by *Neurological Disorders: Public Health Challenges*. The book focused upon public health aspects of the main neurological disorders. The recommendations for action were to strengthen neurological care within existing health systems, incorporate rehabilitation into the

THE WORLD FEDERATION OF NEUROLOGY AND THE WORLD HEALTH ORGANIZATION | **171**

key strategies, develop national capacity and international collaboration, and define priorities for research (4).

In 2009, Benedetto Saraceno retired as head of the WHO Mental Health Office, and Shekhar Saxena succeeded him.

ICD updating

The WHO has the responsibility for the International Classification of Diseases (ICD). In 1982, the WHO consulted the WFN about the revision of the neurological part of the ICD and of the International Nomenclature of Diseases. The WFN objected to the inclusion of cerebrovascular diseases in the cardiovascular chapter rather than in the neurological one. Walter Bradley of Miami and Jean-Marc Orgogozo of Bordeaux gave expert help in the production of a neurological adaptation of ICD-10.

Developments in neurology, with new disease entities, clinical classifications, and considerable progress in diagnosis and treatment of cerebrovascular disorders, necessitated an update, ICD-11. In June 2009, the new ICD-11 Committee was convened in Geneva by Dr Shekhar Saxena and Dr Tarun Dua of the WHO Programme for Neurological Diseases and Neuroscience, Department of Mental Health and Substance Abuse, the WHO division that is responsible for disorders of the nervous system. The committee is very active, and will probably be able to complete the new ICD update in 2015. Raad Shakir, the WFN Secretary-Treasurer General, chairs the Committee (5).

The mental health Gap Action Programme ('mhGAP')

Mental, neurological, and substance abuse disorders are major contributors to morbidity and premature mortality. Fourteen per cent of the global burden of disease, measured in disability-adjusted life years (DALYs) can be attributed to these disorders. In order to reduce the treatment gap and improve services, the WHO launched the mental health Gap Action Programme. WFN is a member of the 'mhGAP Forum' for collaboration and coordinated action (6). This programme has the objective of scaling up care for priority mental, neurological, and substance use disorders especially in low- and middle-income countries.

WFN Public Relations Committee

At the Vancouver congress in 1993, President John Walton established a WFN Public Relations Committee with Professor Donald Paty as Chairman. Due to Professor Paty's health problems, Johan Aarli was invited by John Walton to take over as the new Chairman. Aarli included WHO Liaison Committee matters as its main function, and much of the Committee's work became focused on the effect of the collaboration between the WFN and the WHO, as exampled by the reports on the *Neurology Atlas*, and *Neurological Disorders*.

References

1 **Preamble to the Constitution of the World Health Organization.** In *Basic Documents.* Forty-seventh Edition. WHO Press, Geneva 2009.

2 **Herrman H, Saxena S, Moodle R (Eds).** *Promoting Mental Health: Concepts, Emerging Evidence, Practice.* WHO Press, Geneva 2005.

3 **Saraceno B, Aarli JA, Dua T, Janca A.** *Atlas: Country Resources for Neurological Disorders 2004.* WHO Press, Geneva 2004 (59 pp.).

4 **Saraceno B.** *Neurological Disorders: public health challenges.* WHO Press, Geneva 2006 (218 pp.).

5 **WFN.** WHO take on ICD revisions. *World Neurol* 2009; **24**(5):1,14.

6 **World Health Report 2006.** *Working together for Health.* WHO, Geneva 2006.

Chapter 8

In Service of the World Federation of Neurology

A neurologist remembers Caxias

This section is written by Noshir H. Wadia, Emeritus Director—Department of Neurology, Jaslok Hospital and Research Centre, Mumbai.

My association with the World Federation of Neurology (WFN) coincides with the foundation of the Federation and my returning to India in 1957 with a mandate to develop a department of neurology at my Alma Mater, the Grant Medical College and JJ Hospital, Bombay. Neurology in India was in its infancy then with a handful of neurosurgeons, neurologists, and an even lesser number of neuropathologists and neuroradiologists. Indeed, Indian neurology was recognized abroad because of two stalwart pioneering neurosurgeons who established departments at the medical colleges of South India—Jacob Chandy and B Ramamurthi. In fact, Ramamurthi was the Indian delegate at the Organizational and Constitutional meetings of the World Federation of Neurology, Brussels, Belgium—22 and 26 July 1957.

I am not quite sure how I came to the attention of the WFN. It could be because I was registrar to Russell Brain (Lord Brain) for over four years at two premier Neurological Institutes in London between 1953 and 1957 and published articles in *Brain* soon after. And Russell Brain was amongst the small 'clique' of close friends and associates of Ludo Van Bogaert, who was the leader in the foundation of the WFN (1). Also, William McMenemey and Macdonald Critchley, who were the other associates, knew of me, as I was registrar at the institutes where they were consultants.

Whereas initially the group around Ludo Van Bogaert was essentially European, Americans Houston Merritt and Pearce Bailey, had a major part to play in the foundation of the WFN, having proposed the creation of a World Neurological Federation at a meeting of the American Academy of Neurology in Boston, 1956.

Houston Merritt was a most respected neurologist in the USA and Director of the Neurological Institute of the Columbia Presbyterian Medical Center, New York. And Pearce Bailey was the Director of the newly founded National

Institute of Neurological Diseases and Blindness (NINDB) of the National Institutes of Health (NIH), Bethesda. Indeed it was Pearce Bailey, who was instrumental in obtaining a US government grant of $126,000 per year for five years to establish a secretariat for the infant WFN in Antwerp (1,2). In fact, it was he who chose an American neurologist, Charles Poser, to be the Medical Executive Officer (MEO) of the secretariat under Van Bogaert to keep a close liaison between Americans and Europeans.

One of Charles Poser's assignments was to travel internationally 'to acquaint neurologists in other parts of the World with the general purposes of WFN and enlist their support in getting their respective national neurological associations to join the Federation' (1).

One such visit was in 1959, when Charles Poser and Pearce Bailey came to Bombay, and were impressed with what they saw at the departments of neurology in the two Bombay medical colleges. At that time, I was on the Government of India Committee to enquire into suspected manganese poisoning occurring amongst miners, causing Parkinsonism (3). It could be that Poser's report to Van Bogaert about this research and the fact that I had set up an active department under constraining circumstances, which made Van Bogaert invite me to become a founder member of one of the newly formed Problem Commissions—Tropical Neurology. Its first meeting was held in Buenos Aires, Argentina, 29 November to 2 December 1961, with members of international repute. It was there that I gave a talk on manganese intoxication in Indian mines in the scientific programme of the meeting (4).

Following the meeting, I visited some departments of neurology in Santiago, Chile, and Lima, Peru, the former headed by Oscar Marin, a dynamic young neurologist, and the latter by J O Trelles, a well-known Peruvian neurologist. This was followed by a relaxed stop in Rio de Janeiro, Brazil, on my way back home via Frankfurt. Little did I know what was to follow.

There were very few flights in 1961 to Europe from Rio de Janeiro and I had not closed my return ticket, as I was not sure of how many days I would spend in South America. It was then that I found that seats on the international airlines I wanted were fully booked. I had no choice but to take Panair for Brazil, about which I knew little. Unfortunately, I had not checked what stops it would make. As I was about to board the plane I saw a sign, 'Lisbon'. Believe it or not, I had always intuitively felt that in my travels I should not touch Lisbon or Karachi. India had very unfriendly relations with Portugal and Pakistan and I thought it was best to keep away from them. I was in a dilemma whether to board the plane or turn back. In those days, India had strict foreign exchange regulations and a nominal travel allowance and I had very few dollars left in my pocket to remain in Rio de Janeiro before getting a flight to Frankfurt, which I wanted.

The other option was to go to the Indian Consulate/Embassy and tell them that I was fearful to land on Portuguese soil for a reason that would sound very silly to the Consulate/Embassy officer if all were peaceful there. In 1961 communications were poor across the vast distance between India and South America. No English newspapers were easily available, nor television, and I did not listen to the English radio while I was travelling, which could have alerted me that India had invaded Goa and liberated it from foreign rule.

Finally, I decided to get on board on 19 December hoping that there was no eruption of the simmering trouble between India and Portugal. The flight made a short unscheduled stop at Dakar (Senegal). And on my enquiry whether there was any trouble between our two countries, I was told that there were some of the usual skirmishes, which heightened my apprehension, but I continued my journey. I had no choice. The flight landed in Lisbon late at night and I refused to get off the plane as was requested of all travellers during transit. I could not give any valid reason except that I was intuitively apprehensive to set foot on Portuguese soil. After a couple of hours the transit passengers had not returned, when I realized that something was very wrong and I was the cause of it. A couple of young men in civilian clothes came up and asked me why I was behaving like this, mentioning that the flight had been held up because of me. I had not realized that they were plain-clothes security men and not airline staff. On their persistent request that I should get off the plane and complete transit formalities, I demanded that I wanted to contact the British Ambassador for protection believing that as long as I was in the aeroplane I was on international territory. This request was not granted and in any case it turned out that the British were not representing India. After another hour, two other uniformed men arrived and ordered me to get off the airplane, this time with guns in their hands. My worst fears were confirmed, and I had to get off the plane onto Portuguese soil. Even at that time I did not know that there was a major conflict between our two countries. Finally when I appeared before the immigration police I was told that I was under arrest as there was war between India and Portugal. Telling him that I was a doctor and an innocent bystander did not help. The police chief was very angry with me, pointed to a map and said 'India so large, Goa so small' and Nehru in his opinion was a criminal. I later realized that the building in which I was held at the airport was called, if my memory serves me right, 'Policia Internationale por Defesa do Estado' (International Police for Defence of the State). The immigration formalities, which included photographs of my face and fingerprints, upset me. My passport and belongings were taken away, except for my pyjamas, and I was bundled into a van with grilles, which was obviously a police prisoner vehicle. By this time it was past midnight and I could not see anything in the dark of the city through which I was being driven. It took some time to reach our destination, which was possibly outside Lisbon, and it was obvious that it was a prison with guards, wires, prison cells, etc. I was then pushed into one of the cells and when the door finally closed I realized that I had landed in major trouble. I slouched on to the bed wondering what was going to happen to me—clearly I was a hostage or prisoner of war. It so transpired that I was not alone and there were three other prisoners. Initially I dared not find out who they were. Were they criminals, were they Indians, or were they Portuguese or other foreigners? Finally I had the courage to ask them who they were; they said they were Indians transiting through Lisbon from London on their way to Ghana. They were gold miners from the Kolar Gold fields in India going to gold mines in Ghana, where they were seeking employment. I spent a sleepless night going over the happy days just gone by and, as I wrote to my mother much later, the fall from the top of the Corcovado Mountain in Rio de Janeiro to the depths of a dungeon was shattering.

In the morning I realized that I was in a massive prison, which I later found out was called 'Caxias'; a prison for political dissenters of the dictator Salazar's regime—communists, liberals, or others—and those from Portuguese colonies who had fought against colonial rule. It was only after ten days when another Indian hostage, a doctor, was forced off a Swiss Air flight that we came to know that India had invaded Goa, and that several thousand Portuguese soldiers had been taken prisoner. Our arrest was obviously a reprisal, and we were bargaining chips—totally innocent hostages, possibly some of the first in the world of airplanes.

The cell I was in had a toilet facility, which I shared not only with my three prison inmates but also prisoners from other cells, and for this benefit we were

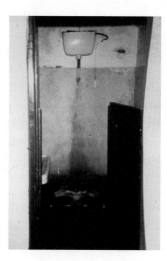

Fig. 8.1 An example of the dirty toilet, which my inmates had to clean, as seen during our later 1992 visit.

Noshir Wadja: Serving the WFN: A Neurologist Remembers Caxias. *World Neurology* Vol. 27, Nos 3 and 4. 2012. Copyright WFN.

ordered to clean the toilet (Fig. 8.1). However, I was spared this task as my inmates respected me as a professional and refused to let me do it, which I accepted reluctantly.

There was a daily routine. In the morning it was coffee with bread and in the afternoon and night rice with bits of fish or meat. It was December and although it was southern Europe, it was bitterly cold. I had only a thin blanket for warmth. And putting my feet into the cold slippers at night to go to the toilet was a chilling experience, which I tried to avoid till the morning. There was no communication with the outside world, except with the guards through gestures, broken English, and a few words of Portuguese I had picked up. We were not let out of the cell for exercise for the first month, and except for the Bible there was nothing to read under the single dim light.

Whilst we were constantly checked even through the night that we had not escaped, and our daily regime was tight, some guards were kind; knowing that I was an innocent badly trapped in this conflict they would quietly slip in an extra pat of butter, a banana, or cigarettes. The world is full of good humans too! My inmates and I often talked about the outcome of this confinement. As they were depressed and occasionally weepy, especially the youngest one who had left his wife and small child in London, I light-heartedly said to keep them cheerful that we should just lie low for six months and then start digging a tunnel. Having not seen the outside of the jail, little did I know that we would be

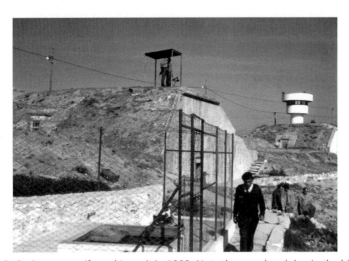

Fig. 8.2 Caxias as my wife and I saw it in 1992. Note the guard and dog in the higher reaches of the prison.

Noshir Wadja: Serving the WFN: A Neurologist Remembers Caxias. *World Neurology* Vol. 27, Nos 3 and 4. 2012. Copyright WFN.

sitting ducks for guards and their dogs looking down from the higher reaches of the prison. This I found out much later.

It was clear that we were in a desperate situation and I began preparing myself for a long stay, but of course I was worried about what was happening at home, to my family, friends, and my department, which I had so carefully nursed. We were never subjected to any torture, but such thoughts were never far away as we could hear cries of others who were being treated more harshly, and maltreatment of hostages in totalitarian regimes was well known. I could not interact in any way with the outside world as we were not allowed to write or given paper to do so in the first month. A Portuguese lawyer, possibly sent through some Jesuit teachers from my old school, came to see me and asked if I wanted to plead for Habeas Corpus. I told him to give me more time to consider the implications of this appeal before the Portuguese court, but later refused. This was because I was advised to do this by another Indian prisoner I had come to know who was a lawyer from Goa in solitary confinement over many years in a cell just across a small passage outside the toilet which separated us. To talk to him I opened the visor in his steel door oiling it with sardine oil to avoid making any noise, whilst my cell mates watched the main corridor outside our cell to warn me about the arrival of guards. The lawyer was taken aback when I spoke in Marathi, a local language, but delighted to hear it. He gave me his name and said he had been in and out of this prison over many years, having been captured for dissidence in Goa and extradited to Lisbon permanently. He said 'if you apply for Habeas Corpus you will be booked for 20 years as they will plant some false evidence to implicate you in a crime or espionage. So keep quiet and patiently wait to see how events unfold'.

One day a guard told me that there was a letter and a parcel sent by Professor Almeida Lima, which was a great surprise. I knew Professor Lima to be a famous Portuguese neurosurgeon because it was he and Egaz Moniz who were first to perform cerebral (carotid artery) angiography and I had bought a book authored by them when I was a trainee in London. I was immensely touched because the parcel contained a sweater, which I was allowed to wear, and some books in English to pass the time. I now recall that one was by Bertrand Russell, which revealed his mind-set. Professor Lima also wrote a letter in which he said that he was distressed and upset that an innocent person like me was incarcerated by his government. He also said that writing this could put him into some trouble, but he did not care. I wish I had kept that letter till today; but I was then a young man in a hurry wanting to get along with life. Obviously, he was not a supporter of Salazar and his government, but there was little he could do about it. It was not possible for me to thank him then because of my situation, but in 1969 at the combined WFN international meeting of

IN SERVICE OF THE WORLD FEDERATION OF NEUROLOGY | **179**

neurologists and neurosurgeons in New York, I got a chance to meet him face to face and profusely thanked him for his kindness and his courage.

After one month we were shifted from the dingy cell to a slightly better prison cell with some bathing facilities, also a pack of cards and cigarettes, which I passed on to my cell mates. I also realized that it was not the British but the Egyptians who had intervened on behalf of India when an Egyptian Consular officer turned up to find out how we were being treated. Nehru and Nasser were great friends!

Along with the Egyptian Consular Officer Shukri Fouad, the Red Cross and Amnesty International were involved in looking after our welfare and release. I am not aware of the role of each of them, but the most concerned were the Egyptian Consular Officer and Amnesty International, which had highlighted our plight in the press. I should also mention here that one of the persons who raised a voice for my release was the late Dr Dorothy Russell, a renowned neuropathologist at the London Hospital, who knew me as a registrar in London. She wrote later after my release in the *British Medical Journal*,

> In December, 1961, Dr N. H. Wadia, an Indian neurologist, well known to many in England having worked as registrar in two London teaching hospitals, was detained in Portugal for two months in the notorious Caxias prison as a reprisal for the Indian annexation of Goa. He had been forcibly removed from a plane in Lisbon while returning from a neurological congress in South America. The first month was spent in a dungeon with another Indian doctor and three Indian engineers, under conditions of deprivation and squalor. Some improvement followed the intervention of the United Arab Republic (the official intermediary between Portugal and India), the Papal Nuncio, and the International Red Cross. Continued pressure from medical bodies and eminent neurologists in this and other European countries, the United States of America, and Chile helped to hasten Dr Wadia's release.
>
> Dr Wadia's experience focuses attention on the work of Amnesty for the plight of the 'forgotten prisoner'. This Society sent a lawyer to Portugal to help him and others amongst whom there were men and women doctors, of whose imprisonment they had learnt. . . . (5).

The elderly Indian doctor, who had a cardiac ailment, was released at the end of a month on health grounds through the intervention of the Red Cross. But the three gold miners and I had to wait another month when, on 20 February 1962, we were suddenly told that we were to be set free. No explanation was given. I was taken to a hotel and next day put on a flight to London where I was greeted by well wishers, and soon returned back to Bombay into the arms of my family and a host of admiring students who had come to the airport (Fig. 8.3 and Fig. 8.4).

After release I came to know that friends and concerned colleagues in the UK had heard of our capture and some accounts and protests appeared in the newspapers there. My mother and brothers though worried that I had not returned

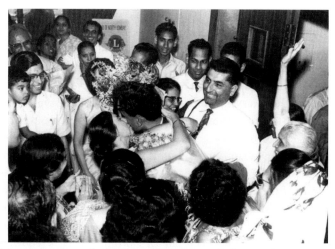

Fig. 8.3 A warm welcome by family and friends on arrival at Bombay airport.

Noshir Wadja: Serving the WFN: A Neurologist Remembers Caxias. *World Neurology* Vol. 27, Nos 3 and 4. 2012. Copyright WFN.

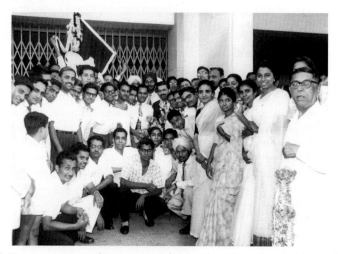

Fig. 8.4 Upon my return, I also was greeted at Bombay airport by admiring undergraduate students of the Grant Medical College and JJ Hospital.

Noshir Wadja: Serving the WFN: A Neurologist Remembers Caxias. *World Neurology* Vol. 27, Nos 3 and 4. 2012. Copyright WFN.

were not aware for some days of my predicament. This was because there was no fixed date for my return and communications in those days were not easy and the Indian Government had not contacted them. They were shocked when the influential wife of the doctor, who was subsequently captured, informed them about my arrest. After this my brother Jimmy remained in New Delhi for a month pleading with whomever he could, including Jawaharlal Nehru, for my release. His experience with the Government is another story.

I was told that we had not been exchanged for Portuguese soldiers held prisoner in Goa. The three miners were released through the intervention of the Pope because they were Catholics and Salazar was devout. I remember that they had asked for a Mass in the prison and were permitted to have it. As for me, I heard from a very reliable source that there was intervention on my behalf by some well-wishers of Indian origin from one of the African Portuguese colonies who had the confidence of Salazar and my exchange was for an iconic 400-year-old statue of Jesus Christ enshrined in a Goa Church which Salazar wanted. I have never been able to fully confirm this information from any other source but am humbled if true.

Somehow I did not feel bitter or dejected and thanked God it was all over. And soon I was back to my old duties developing my department. Later in the year I flew to Tokyo to participate in the first Asian Oceanian Congress of Neurology October 7–10 1962 organized by the WFN. As we skirted China in the Air India plane, I wondered if fate would force me to land there, as by then India and China were having major border conflicts. And indeed war broke out on 20 October 1962!

I must complete this story about Portugal with two very pleasant subsequent experiences, which have left fond memories of that country and its people. The first was a visit with my wife as a tourist in 1992. At that time we paid a courtesy call to the Indian ambassador to whom we had been introduced. During the conversation he asked if this was our first visit to Portugal and whilst I was not sure what to say, my wife said 'it is my first visit and his second' and she mentioned my experience of Lisbon in 1961–1962. The ambassador was taken aback and could just recall some details of these events, as he must have been a young officer then; and he said he could arrange a visit to the prison, as relations between Portugal and India were very cordial. My wife was most keen to do this and I was ready, as I carried no wounds to reopen. My wife to whom I was not married when I was a prisoner could not believe that an innocent person had been thrown in a dungeon and not kept in a more acceptable environment under house arrest. This time the experience was most pleasant as we were special guests of Caxias. We were driven on a sunny day through the streets of Lisbon and the prison did not seem too far. We were met by the Superintendent of the prison and escorted by a translator who spoke English (Fig. 8.5). The superintendent, a young man who was probably a boy in 1961 was very surprised and asked what crime had I committed when we recalled my days of imprisonment for him. The first area we visited was nothing like the description I had given my wife of where I was initially lodged. This was possibly where I spent the second

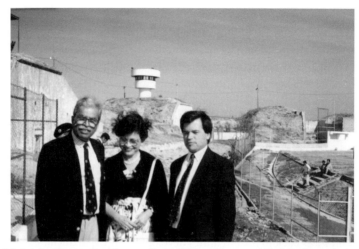

Fig. 8.5 I visited Portugal with my wife in 1992, where we visited Caxias and met the young superintendent of the prison (on the right).

Noshir Wadja: Serving the WFN: A Neurologist Remembers Caxias. *World Neurology* Vol. 27, Nos 3 and 4. 2012. Copyright WFN.

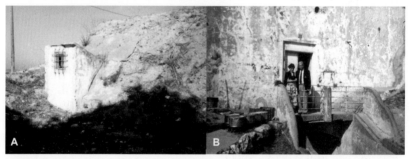

Fig. 8.6 The photo on the left shows the outside of the dilapidated dungeon where I was confined as seen in 1992. On the right, my wife and I stand outside a prison door in 1992.

Noshir Wadja: Serving the WFN: A Neurologist Remembers Caxias. *World Neurology* Vol. 27, Nos 3 and 4. 2012. Copyright WFN.

month. I told the Superintendent that I was definitely not in this kind of prison but in one much worse. He then took us to the back of the large complex where the remains of the old prison stood which convinced my wife of my harrowing experience. (Fig. 8.6)

We ended this visit in the Superintendent's office with a toast in fine Port wine to Portugal and India's friendship. At that time I was given a memento of a wall plate of Caxias made by the then prisoners and a set of coasters.

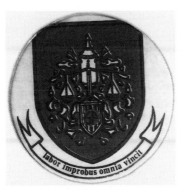

Fig. 8.7 This is a photograph of a coaster made by the prisoners, which the prison superintendent gave to my wife and I as a memento of our 1992 visit.

Noshir Wadja: Serving the WFN: A Neurologist Remembers Caxias. *World Neurology* Vol. 27, Nos 3 and 4. Copyright WFN.

The other occasion was in April 1994 when I was invited to participate in the 3rd International Workshop on Machado-Joseph Disease (SCA3), sponsored by the WFN at San Miguel in the very beautiful island of Azores, where I presented my research paper on a subject of mutual interest—Olivopontocerebellar Atrophy with Slow Eye Movements (SCA2). I met several Portuguese neurologists researching hereditary ataxias and told them of my earlier experience in their country and how pleasant it was to be back under totally different circumstances. Not so old as I, their memory of Salazar was rather distant although they were aware of their country's history.

There are several incidents and anecdotes some funny and some more serious, which I have not mentioned because they are not relevant to my association with the WFN, which I may expand on some day. In the successive years I involved myself with various research groups and committees of the WFN and in 1989 was elected as Vice President of the WFN. All this has left very pleasant memories of my 50 years of service with the WFN, on which I can look back in my retirement with contentment.

What I have written is entirely from my own memory of events, and there may be errors in small details, as I have never kept diaries of my life. Yet, constant recall over the years has left an indelible imprint somewhat mellowed by advanced age.

Internal Political Struggle in Kyoto

This section is written by Jun Kimura.

The Vancouver World Congress of Neurology preceded the International Congress of EEG and Clinical Neurophysiology organized by the International Federation of Clinical Neurophysiology (IFCN), which I served as President at that time. In retrospect, this occasion marked the beginning of my WFN career although, in those days, I had no intention or ambition to play any political role for the cause of neurology. I wanted to work only in the area of clinical neurophysiology for which I always had a soft spot in my heart.

As the time of the subsequent WFN election approached, the Nominating Committee, headed by Professor Eero Hokkanen from Helsinki, began to look for potential candidates for the Executive Committee outside the traditionally strong North America and Europe, which, in effect, had monopolized the office since its inception. To make the organization more global, Dr Frank Yatsu, a member of the Committee, apparently asked Dr Eijiro Satoyoshi, then one of the Regional Vice Presidents, to recommend someone from Asia in general and Japan in particular, which had participated very actively in the affairs of the WFN. Although I was totally unaware, my name must have surfaced in the process probably from sources close to the IFCN, the only international organization that I had served with any consistency.

Professor Hokkanen came to Kyoto for a sight-seeing tour in 1995 and, in passing, asked if he could have a chance to chat with me. I went to the Grand Hotel near Kyoto station to see him not knowing to what this pertained. After a very brief pleasantry, he asked if I would be interested in the office of the President, which was a big surprise. But I managed to tell him I would not run for the top position without prior experience in the Executive Committee of the WFN, which I had known only for a couple of years as a member of the Public Relations Committee. Nothing much happened and I more or less forgot about this brief encounter.

In 1996, Dr Yatsu came to Japan to persuade the Japanese Society of Neurology to nominate me for the position of First Vice President. After a brief discussion at the Board of Directors meeting, Dr Thoru Mannen, then the Chairman of the Japanese Society of Neurology, formally announced my candidacy, a signal that surprised many WFN insiders as an unprecedented deviation from the traditional candidacy. As I was totally unknown in the neurological community, most delegates initially thought this bid had no serious merit. But, I felt I might have a fighting chance if I could mobilize my neurophysiology friends globally to campaign on my behalf. Otherwise, I would not have run.

While I was preparing for the election, I had to face a totally unexpected personal crisis. This turn of events climaxed with a sadly misdirected legal prying into my bank accounts used for a drug trial of botulinum toxin and for fund-raising to organize the 1995 Kyoto International Congress of EMG and Clinical Neurophysiology. One of my close associates working with me in the Department of Neurology was detained while I was abroad attending a Brazilian EMG workshop organized by my friend Dr Joao Nobrege. On my return to Japan, 200 reporters

IN SERVICE OF THE WORLD FEDERATION OF NEUROLOGY | **185**

surrounded me, wanting to capture the moment of arrest which, however, did not materialize. To this date, I do not know exactly what happened but I assume that the prosecutor's office quickly realized that they had made a false accusation. In the meantime, Dr Hiroshi Shibasaki, a good friend of mine and an internationally known neurophysiologist, alerted, by e-mail, many friends of mine worldwide, who, in turn, sent more than 100 letters of protest to the prosecutor's office that I had endured an unjustifiable legal probe without due cause.

As the news, carried by CNN and other media, reached the WFN headquarters, I received a letter from President Lord John Walton, who expressed concern as to whether I would be an acceptable candidate for a high office in the midst of this turmoil. Fortunately, by then, I was able to reply that the incident, widely publicized as one of the biggest scandals of the year, ended happily (for us) with the resignation of the chief prosecutor in the Kyoto office and disbandment of the special force created to incriminate us. My associate, after the maximal detention period of 21 days, also came out of prison triumphantly, proving yet again that justice may be blind but the truth always sets you free. In passing, I should mention that in the Osaka high court, which oversaw the Kyoto office, the malicious prosecution triggered an internal power struggle, leading to the arrest of the Director of Public Safety Commission, who single-handedly objected to the mishandling of the legal probe in our case and to subsequent attempts to cover up. While in jail, he published a 300-page prison memoire, exposing all of his former colleagues, including the chief prosecutor, who supported our arrest on bribery charges despite evidence to the contrary, and prolonged investigation as a face-saving manoeuvre, even when he realized they had no case.

This outcome strengthened my position as a legitimate candidate for WFN office as the unintended publicity worked to my advantage in international politics. Thus, I was elected as First Vice President during the 1997 Buenos Aires Congress. While the votes were counted during the session, one of the delegates from Latin America approached and said 'I am very happy that you broke out of the jail just in time for this election!' Despite such sentiment, which prevailed, members of the Council of Delegates received me warmly, once they realized that I was an innocent victim. I was very happy to serve the WFN in this capacity, a position created anew in 1997. During the previous fiscal periods, the Chairman of the Research Committee also held the Office of the First Vice Presidency, having dual functions, perhaps with an excessive burden of responsibilities and commitment of time.

Acknowledgements

Noshir H. Wadia: thanks are due to the superintendent of Caxias in 1992 for permission to photograph and have photographs taken without reservation.

It was a demonstration of heart-warming cordiality. To the Indian Ambassador for arranging the revival visit for my wife and I, and erstwhile President of the WFN Professor Johan Aarli for stimulating me to write this account for the first time, as earlier I felt it was too personal to be of interest to anyone. He believed that this would be worth a mention in his history of the WFN, which he is writing. Finally, my elder brother Jimmy without whose effort to get me released I would have remained longer in Caxias or suffered a worse fate, as also for the airport photographs.

References

1 **Poser CM.** The World Federation of Neurology: the formative period 1955–1961. Personal recollections. *J Neurol Sci* 1993; **120**: 218–27.

2 **Walton J.** The WFN comes of age. *J Neurol Sci* 2008; **268**: 1–5.

3 **Report of Manganese Poisoning Enquiry Committee.** Ministry of Labour and Employment, Government of India 1960.

4 **Wadia NH.** Manganese Intoxication in Indian mines. In: Bogaert LV, Kafer JP, Poch GF, editors. Tropical Neurology—Proceedings of the first International Symposium held in Buenos Aires, November 29-2 December 1961 organised by WFN and Sociedad Neurologica Argentina Buenos Aires. Lopez Libreros Editores S.R.L. 1961; 271–77.

5 This article was first published in an abbreviated form in *World Neurology* 2012 for the book on the history of the WFN. In 2012, I became the editor-in-Chief of *World Neurology*. Professor Noshir Wadia, Mumbai, India, President Vladimir Hachinski, WFN, Peter Bakker, and Jeff Evans as managing editor on behalf of Elsevier, and I gave joint permission to publish the story. Part 1 appeared as 'A founder of contemporary Indian neurology details the events of his imprisonment in Portugal'. Volume 27(3), June 2012, 8–10. Part 2 appeared as 'The second and final part of Dr Wadia's remarkable story about his imprisonment in Portugal'. Volume 27(4), August 2012, 10–11.

6 **Poser CM.** The World Federation of Neurology: the formative period 1955–1961. Personal recollections. *J Neurol Sci* 1993; **120**: 218–27.

7 **Walton J.** The WFN comes of age. *J Neurol Sci* 2008; **268**: 1–5.

8 **Report of Manganese Poisoning Enquiry Committee.** Ministry of Labour and Employment, Government of India 1960.

9 **Wadia NH.** Manganese Intoxication in Indian mines. In: Bogaert LV, Käfer JP, Poch GF, editors. Tropical Neurology—Proceedings of the first International Symposium held in Buenos Aires, November 29-2 December 1961 organized by WFN and Sociedad Neurologica Argentina, Buenos Aires. Lopez Libreros Editores S.R.L. 1993; 271–77.

10 **Amulree, Bywaters EGL, Collier J, Russell DS.** 'Amnesty'. Correspondence. *Br Med J* 19 May 1962; **1**: 1418.

Chapter 9

The International (World) Congresses of Neurology

How were the Congress venues selected?

The World Federation of Neurology (WFN) was founded in Brussels in 1957, during the 6th International Neurological Congress. It was also called the First International Congress of Neurological Sciences because it was much more comprehensive in neurosciences than the previous five congresses had been. The Third International Congress of Neuropathology, the Fifth Symposium of Neuroradiology, the Fifth Meeting of the International League against Epilepsy, and the Fourth International Congress of Electroencephalography and Clinical Neurophysiology also took place in Brussels simultaneously. And for the first time there was an International Congress of Neurosurgery. Ludo van Bogaert was the Secretary General of the Congress.

All participants wore a badge comprising an identification label (name and country) and a ribbon, the colour of which varied according to the discipline of the bearer: neurology, yellow; neuropathology, orange; neurosurgery, red; electroencephalography, blue; and neuroradiology, green. The International League Against Epilepsy (ILAE) used to have their meetings about the time and place of the International Neurological Congresses. In 1973, this was changed to state that the International Congress of the League 'shall be held ordinarily each 4 years at about the time and at or near the place of the International Congress of Neurology' (1). In 1957, the place was Brussels. Brussels became the Neurosciences Fair in 1957.

The first international congress of neurology, in which the WFN was directly engaged in the preparations, was the Seventh International Neurological Congress, which took place in Rome in September 1961. The first six congresses are discussed in Chapter 1. They have no direct connection with the Federation, simply because there was no WFN at that time. However, many of the key persons who convened had already attended several of the preceding post-war congresses of neurology.

In 1961, the WFN was well established. The organization had an administration, a constitution, and an economy. The number of member societies had increased. The new elements—the Problem Commissions—were focusing upon central research topics in international neurology.

In his Presidential Report during the International Congress of Neurology in Vienna in 1965, Ludo van Bogaert was concerned about the preparation of the future congress programmes. It was his hope to create a permanent organization, which would establish continuity and tradition in the organization of world congresses of neurology. He was very clear that the WFN Problem Commissions—later renamed Research Committees—should have a central function in deciding the scientific programmes.

> The congresses are still being organized according to a rather ill defined tradition, inherited from the old international congresses, where individual influences and local obligations from the host country still predominate. The WFN had hoped that the Executive Committee and the selection of major topics had approved once the selection of a host country and topic directors had been made, that the topic directors before inviting qualified rapporteurs could have taken advantage of the competency of the Problem Commissions. It is the latter who actually have the ability to designate at a given moment the most qualified investigators in a particular field (2).

And who selected them?

At the previous international congresses of neurology, representatives from various national neurological associations met during the congress and discussed where the next congress should take place. When this was decided, the local organizing committee was relatively free to organize the programme.

The World Congresses of Neurology dominate events in neurology. But a Congress is only a Neuroscience Fair. The WFN is the dynamo, in continuous activity between the Congresses, guarding the responsibilities for the development of international neurology.

When the WFN was established, the Council of Delegates of the Federation met during the congress, evaluated bids from various neurological societies for the next congress venues, and presented proposals for the scientific programme, such as possible topics and rapporteurs. The venue was chosen after a ballot, and there was thus a partnership between the WFN on the one hand and the chosen host society. This agreement was followed until the Amsterdam Congress 1977.

Van Bogaert proposed '1) to reorganize all the specialized neurologic disciplines along the central axis of neurology by investing them in a coordinated program, which would allocate two days for major topics of common interest to all the constituent groups and two days for independent sessions of each participating discipline, and 2) to reduce to a minimum the time allocated for free communications' (3).

A new policy was established from Amsterdam (1977) onwards. The WFN assumed the responsibility for choosing the venue for the subsequent World Congress of Neurology, and identified the main issues of the programme. Local organizing and scientific advisory committees were selected, and the Federation and the committees therefore now had close contact during the preparation of the final programme.

International Travelling around 1960

Travelling to an international congress before World War II, with the usual journey by sea across the Atlantic, might take about five days. Air travel now has cut that down to about half a day or less. Scheduled jet flights began in October 1958, which was the first year when more people crossed the Atlantic by plane than by ship.

The political development in the post-war era led to a rise in commercial cooperation between western European countries and the USA. This also increased tourism and made air travel easier. International permits and civil aviation acts, long runways, and technological developments, such as the advent of the Boeing 707, were key factors in the expansion of commercial air travel.

The 7th International Neurological Congress—the Second International Congress of Neurology (Rome 1961)

President, Mario Gozzano; Secretary-General, Giovanni Alema; Vice President, H. Houston Merritt.

The decision that Rome should be the congress venue was made in Brussels, before the WFN had been established. The Congress was held under the auspices of the WFN and of the NINDB the main sponsor of the congress. The American Joint Committee on International Affairs was strongly involved in the organization of the meeting and it was not only a neurology Congress. It also became the Fifth International Congress of Electroencephalography and Clinical Neurophysiology (4).

Prior to 1973, ILAE Conferences were not officially numbered, but simply called 'ILAE Meetings'. The Rome ILAE Meeting took place on 7–13 September, and the WFN Congress on 10–15 September. Although the neurosurgeons and neuropathologists had their own meetings, many neuropathologists arrived in Rome from the neuropathology conference in Munich that closed immediately before the Rome meeting. Some of the WFN Problem Commissions had taken the opportunity to organize separate meetings on neurological geography, on the history of neurology, on multiple sclerosis, and on neuroradiology. The WFN Problem Commission on the history of neurology had had their meeting at Varennes in the north-east of France, and the guests came to Rome from Varennes. Nearly 1500 participants attended the congress. The Berlin Wall was built in 1960, but no one from East Germany was allowed to travel.

Honorary Presidents at the Rome congress were Sir Gordon Holmes, Georges Guillain, André-Thomas, Théophile Alajouanine, Antonio Flores, Georg H. Monrad-Krohn, Knud Krabbe, Henry A. Riley, and Paul van Gehuchten.

The scientific sessions were held in the Palazzo Pio on the Vatican side of the river. The topics were neurological disorders in porphyria, phenylketonuria, and galactosuria, and neurological disorders related to liver diseases. The second day was dedicated to brain disturbances associated with cardio-pulmonary disorders, and the third day to aphasia.

Houston Merritt chaired the sessions on neurological disorders in porphyria, phenylketonuria, and galactosuria, and on neurological disorders related to liver disease. Gustav Bodechtel conducted the session on brain disturbances associated with cardio-pulmonary disease. The session on aphasia was conducted by Macdonald Critchley, who also pointed out that 1961 was the centenary of Henry Head's birth, and also of Paul Broca's first contribution to neurosciences.

The registration fee amounted to US$15; banquet and evening dance $11 (not included). The social programme included receptions at the Diocletian Baths, the Capitoline Museum, and at the Castello San Angelo. His Holiness Pope John held a private audience for members of the congress at the Castello Gondolfo.

According to the WFN constitution and bye-laws, the WFN President and the Secretary-Treasurer General should each serve for four years. A meeting of the national representatives of the WFN took place at the end of the congress, and Ludo van Bogaert and Pearce Bailey were unanimously re-elected for a second term. Houston Merritt (New York) and Raymond Garcin (Paris) were elected Vice Presidents.

The 8th International Congress of Neurology—the Third International Congress of Neurology (Vienna 1965)

President: Hans Hoff; Secretary-General: Helmuth Tschabitscher; Vice President Franz Seitelberger.

The 8th International Congress of Neurology took place in Vienna on 5–10 September 1965 at the Palais Palffy. The Executive Committee (Council of Delegates) met in the Palais Palffy the day before, 4 September. Thirty-five WFN national delegates met, some of them also representing additional WFN member societies by proxy. Karl Leonhard from Charité, Jochen Quandt from a regional hospital in Bernburg, and Dagobert Mülle (Charité) represented the East German neurologists. Unfortunately, President Ludo van Bogaert was unable to attend because of illness, and Macdonald Critchley read his report. Macdonald Critchley was elected the new President of the WFN, and Henry Miller became Secretary-Treasurer General. The main topics at the congress were sequelae of head injuries, diagnostics of atrophies and muscular hypertrophy, myasthenia gravis, and clinical electromyography. The congress fee was US$30.

The 6th International Congress of Electroencephalography and the meeting of the ILAE and the International Bureau against Epilepsy (IBE) were organized together with the International Congress of Neurology. There was at that time considerable internal discussion among the EEGers whether electromyography should be included in clinical neurophysiology. At that time, the idea of welding all the various branches of clinical neurophysiology into a single federation did not have universal appeal (5).

The 9th International Congress of Neurology—the Fourth International Congress of Neurological Sciences (New York 1969)

President, H. Houston Merritt; Secretary-General, Melvin D. Yahr; Treasurer, Morris B. Bender.

The next congress took place in New York, and it was the first international neurology congress to be organized outside of Europe. The congress venue was the Hilton Hotel, and it was held during 20–27 September. At the Council of Delegates, Macdonald Critchley and Henry Miller were re-elected for a second period.

When it became known in advance that the next Neurological Congress would be in the USA, the General Assembly of the IFCN had agreed to leave the place and time of the EEG Congress to the American EEG Society 'provided that the time should be close to that of the International Neurology Congress'. Thus began the relative independence of the neurology and the EEG congresses that has been maintained ever since (5). This was the 11th ILAE/IBE Congress.

The 4th International Congress of Neurological Surgery was organized simultaneously with the Neurology Congress. Earl Walker was the President of the Neurosurgery Congress, Collin S. MacCarthy the Secretary, and J. Lawrence Pool the Treasurer. There were combined meetings of the two congresses devoted to the major themes of the epilepsies, and of cerebral vascular disorders.

The major themes of the individual sessions and the free communication of the neurology congress included cerebral dominance, nutritional and metabolic disorders of the nervous system, and geographic and viral disorders of the nervous system.

The Fulton Society, the International Multiple Sclerosis Society, and the ILAE also held their meetings in New York during the two congresses while the 7th International Congress of Electroencephalography and Clinical Neurophysiology was held at El Cortez Hotel (temporarily re-named El Cortex) in San Diego the week before. The San Diego congress also marked the occasion of Hans Berger's first paper on EEG (5).

The neurosurgeons had their banquet at the Hilton on 24 September, and the neurologists the following night, 25 September. An opera performance was held at the new opera house in the Lincoln Center on 23 September.

The 10th International Congress of Neurology—the Fifth International Congress of Neurology (Barcelona 1973)

President, A. Subirana; Secretary-General, J.M. Espadaler Medina; Vice President, I. Barraquer Bordas.

The congress took place in the modern Barcelona Congress Centre. The main topics were iatrogenic neurological processes, tropical neurology, transmissible and genetical dementias, and myasthenia gravis and myasthenic syndromes. There was a symposium on current trends in Parkinson's research on 15 September, and the International Federation of Multiple Sclerosis met on 12 September. The 12th ILAE/IBE Congress took place on 8–10 September.

Sigvald Refsum was unanimously elected President of the WFN. He chose Professor Bent de Fine Olivarius of Aarhus, Denmark, as his Secretary-Treasurer General. Olivarius had, however, health problems, and Professor Palle Juul-Jensen, also of Aarhus, soon had to take over due to Dr Olivarius' illness.

The 11th International Congress of Neurology—the Sixth International Congress of Neurology (Amsterdam 1977)

President, W. A. Den Hartog Jager; Secretary-General, George Bruyn; Treasurer-General, A.P.J. Heijstee.

The first neurology congresses were named International Congresses of Neurology. Since Amsterdam 1977, they have been called World Congresses of Neurology. The role of the WFN was now better defined, and at the Council of

THE INTERNATIONAL (WORLD) CONGRESSES OF NEUROLOGY | **193**

Delegates at the end of the congress, proposals were discussed about possible themes, topics, and rapporteurs who should contribute to, and organize, the scientific programme. The Dutch Society of Neurology and the WFN were responsible for the congress.

From then on, the WFN became responsible for choosing the venue for the subsequent World Congresses. National neurological societies had been invited to come up with bids. The bids were presented to the Council of Delegates, who decided the venue on the basis of their attractiveness. The winner organized the local organizing committee, which met with the WFN two years before the congress.

As soon as it was known that the World Congress of Neurology would take place in Amsterdam, it was clear that the 9th EEG congress should precede that of the ILAE the week before (5). This was the 13th ILAE Congress/9th IBE Symposium. Sigvald Refsum was re-elected as President for another four years.

At the Amsterdam congress in 1977, it was recommended that the WFN Research Committee should be consulted regarding the topics for the Congress, and that it should play an active role in planning the scientific programme of the Congress. It was also recommended that the Research Groups be encouraged to hold meetings in temporal and geographical relationship to the Congress.

Three countries were suggested for the 12th World Congress of Neurology in 1981: Czechoslovakia, Kenya, and Japan. The delegates voted by ballot: 35 voted for Japan, nine for Czechoslovakia and eight for Kenya. It was agreed that the congress venue would be Kyoto and Dr Tadeo Tsubaki thanked the Council of Delegates on behalf of the Japanese Society and Japan.

The 12th World Congress of Neurology—the Seventh International Congress of Neurology (Kyoto 1981)

President, S. Katsuki; Secretary General, Tadao Tsubaki.

This was the first World Congress of Neurology to be held in the eastern hemisphere. It was held at the International Congress Centre in Kyoto, Japan, and was remarkably successful. More than 2600 participants from 69 countries were present. From now on, congress enumeration followed the established system, including the congresses from 1931.

The 10th International Congress of Electroencephalography and Clinical Neurophysiology and the Symposium of the International Bureau for Epilepsy took place at the same centre on 12–18 September, followed by the 14th World Congress of the International League Against Epilepsy.

The main topics were hemispheric specialization in man, cerebral vascular diseases, neurotransmitter and neuropeptide dysfunction in relation to neurological disease, and viral infections of the nervous system.

The Congress earned a profit of DM18,000.

Five Vice Presidents were elected, who were also Associate Editors: Shaul Feldman (Israel), Irena Hausmanowa-Petrusewicz (Poland), Ernesto Herskovits (Argentina), Hirotaro Narabayashi (Japan), and J. Manuel Martinez-Lage (Spain).

The 13th World Congress of Neurology (Hamburg 1985)

President, Klaus Poeck; General Secretary, H-G. Mertens; Vice President, Professor H. Gänshirt.

The Congress was held in the Congress Centre and the Plaza hotel at the botanical gardens near the centre of Hamburg. H. Bauer (Göttingen), R. Jung (Freiburg), and Klaus-Joachim Zülch (Köln) were Honorary Presidents.

The main themes were brain and behaviour, ageing and the dementias, neuroimaging, and neuroepidemiology and clinical trials.

This was the first World Congress of Neurology attended by the Pan African Association of Neurological Sciences (PAANS) as an organization.

It was agreed in Hamburg that individual subscriptions paid by members of the WFN Research Groups to funds of the WFN Research Committee in Geneva should be continued. The only grants received by the Research Committee over the last two years had been of the order of US$250 through the International Federation of Multiple Sclerosis (now acting as RG for MS) and $500 from the Third World Medical Research Foundation.

It was accepted at the Hamburg congress that the WFN would be given a proportion of the profits made by the world congress. This decision became important for the future world congresses.

There were 2232 participants at the Hamburg Congress, which was exceptionally well covered by the new newsletter *World Neurology*. The first issue covered the meeting of the Council of Delegates and Research Committee in June 1983.

The 14th World Congress of Neurology (New Delhi 1989)

President, Eddie P. Bharucha; Secretary-General, Jagjit Chopra.

The congress was held on 22–27 October in the Taj Palace, New Delhi. There were 2114 active participants. The Council of Delegates was held on 25 October. The 18th International Epilepsy Congress took place immediately before, and a common session was held on the afternoon of 21 October and forenoon of 22 October.

The first WFN endowed lecture was given in New Delhi. It was made possible by a grant to the WFN from Victor and Clara Soriano. Professor Albert J. Aguayo (Montreal) presented the Soriano Lecture during the World Congress in New Delhi in 1989. The symposium during which the Soriano Lecture takes place is now known as the Fulton Society Symposium.

In New Delhi, John Walton was elected President of the WFN. Frank Clifford Rose was elected Secretary-Treasurer General, and James Toole succeeded George W. Bruyn as Editor-in-Chief of the *Journal of the Neurological Sciences*. It was decided that the WFN should give interest-free loans to support congresses, it would share in any profit on a 50% basis. When no loans were involved in sponsorship, the share given to the WFN would be only 10% of the profits.

According to the constitution, the surplus of the New Delhi Congress could not be taken out of India. The congress did generate a substantial profit, but under Indian government regulations, the money could not be transferred to central funds of the WFN, but had to stay in India to support activities sponsored by the Federation in that country. Fifty per cent of it would be disposed of by the WFN, and 50% by the organizing society.

The 15th World Congress of Neurology (Vancouver 1993)

President, Henry Barnett; Secretary- General, Donald W. Paty; Chairman, Scientific Program Committee, Alberto Aguayo.

The congress took place at the Convention Centre 5–10 September 1993. There were 3400 delegates attending the congress. There were four days of whole day symposia devoted to the major themes of (1) molecular mechanisms of neurologic disease, (2) headache, (3) neural degeneration and regeneration, and (4) environmental neurology. There were 38 symposia and workshops, eight early morning lectures, and four forums for debate. Stanley Prusiner, Nobel Laureate 1997, gave one of the introductory lectures on molecular mechanisms when he spoke about prion diseases. The topic for the presidential symposium on 9 September was Prevention of Stroke: Progress in Primary and Secondary Measures.

The symposium during which the Soriano Lecture takes place is known as the Fulton Society Symposium. At the Fulton Society Symposium on 6 September, Professor Rita Levi-Montalcini (Rome) gave the Soriano Lecture on 'The Modulatory Role of NGF in the Nervous, Endocrine and Immune Systems'. Richard Johnson gave the Victor and Clara Soriano Lecture on the opening day, 6 September, on 'Emerging Infections of the Nervous System'.

The International Congress of Electroencephalography and Clinical Neurophysiology preceded the World Congress. Jun Kimura served as President at the EEG congress. In retrospect, this occasion marked the beginning of his WFN career although, in those days, he had no intention or ambition to play any political role for the cause of neurology.

Lord Walton was re-elected WFN President, Klaus Poeck First Vice President, Frank Clifford Rose Secretary-Treasurer General, and James Toole Editor-in-Chief of the *Journal of the Neurological Sciences*.

Five Vice Presidents were elected: Henry Barnett (Canada), Armand Lowenthal (Belgium), A. Rascol (France), A. Pinelli (Italy), and Eijiro Satoyoshi (Japan). Vladimir Hachinski was elected Chairman of the Steering Committee, and Robert Daroff, the Chairman of the Finance Committee.

Seven national neurological societies applied for the location of the 1997 World Congress, and the Council of Delegates decided that it should take place in Buenos Aires, Argentina.

The 16th World Congress of Neurology (Buenos Aires 1997)

President, Salomon Muchnik; Secretary, Leonor Gold; Treasurer, Lorenzo Bauso Toselli; Chairman of the Scientific Programme Committee, Roberto Sica.

This was the largest WFN Congress so far, with 5200 attendees. The Congress took place on 14–19 September 1997. Roger N. Rosenberg (Dallas) gave the Soriano Lecture on 'The Future of Gene Therapy for Neurological Disease'. Acute stroke was a main theme, and Werner Hacke reviewed the evidence for a therapeutic window in acute stroke. Epilepsy, another major issue, received considerable attention, and Edward Reynolds outlined the Global Campaign Against Epilepsy, a campaign particularly concerned with developing countries, and Amadou Gallo Diop discussed the difficulties facing epilepsy sufferers in developing countries. Dementia was also a central theme, and Mangone reviewed selected Latin-American surveys to evaluate the public health strategies to cope with the anticipated increased number of elderly with cognitive impairment.

For the Buenos Aires congress, Congresos Internacionales was the commercial organizing company.

At most previous World Congresses, there have been no contenders for the Office of President. The only exception was in New Delhi 1989, when John Walton was elected. In Buenos Aires, the Nominating Committee had agreed unanimously with the Council of Delegates to recommend five candidates for the office of WFN President: Jagjit Chopra, Franz Gerstenbrand, James Lance, Klaus Poeck, and James F. Toole. There were also five candidates for the First Vice-Presidency: Antonio Culebras, Franz Gerstenbrand, Jun Kimura, F. Rubio Donnadieu, and James Toole. At the elections, James Toole was elected WFN President, Jun Kimura First Vice President, and Frank Clifford Rose Secretary-Treasurer General (to 31 December 1998).

The 17th World Congress of Neurology (London, UK 2001)

President, Ian McDonald; Secretary-General, Christopher Kennard; Secretary-Treasurer, Richard Godwin-Austen; Chairman of the Scientific Programme Committee, Richard A. C. Hughes.

The first choice of venue for the London Congress had been London's Barbican Centre. The record number of participants at the Buenos Aires Congress led the organizing committee to move the venue to Earls Court, which was not available in November. The congress therefore took place on 17–22 June 2001 and was attended by over 6700 participants from 111 countries.

The London Congress was a historic meeting, because it marked the formal dissolution of the old organization and the transfer of the finances and other assets to the incorporated WFN, which had co-existed alongside its namesake for the past three years.

Since the World Congress took place in the UK, there was no EFNS congress that year. The participants were welcomed by Professor Ian McDonald as WFN Congress President, WFN President James F Toole, EFNS President Jes Olesen, and Charles Warlow as the President of the Association of British Neurologists. The Regimental Band of the Coldstream Guards played during the opening ceremony and then led a procession of presidents and delegates through to a reception in the exhibition hall.

The five main themes were stroke, dementia, epilepsy, multiple sclerosis, and neuromuscular disease. Martin Rossor gave the inaugural Macdonald Critchley Lecture on the early diagnosis of Alzheimer's disease. Stanley Fahn gave the Marsden Memorial Lecture on Dystonia. These were new endowed lectures that were only given at the London congress.

Two new endowed lectures appeared for the first time at the London congress, both named after central figures in the history of the WFN. The World Neurology Foundation sponsored both. Timothy Pedley gave The Richard L. and Mary Masland Lecture on 'Epilepsy—New Therapeutic Developments'. Donald Calne gave The Melvin Yahr Lecture on 'Parkinsonian Disease: Acquired or Inherited'. Melvin Yahr served as Chairman of the Department of Neurology at

Mount Sinai Hospital from 1973 to 1992, and was a world leader in introducing L-dopa treatment for Parkinson's disease.

Francis Collins (USA) gave the Victor and Clara Soriano Award Lecture: 'The Human Genome Project'. Olle Lindvall (Sweden) gave the Soriano Lecture: 'Transplantation in Clinical Practice'.

The Neurological Tournament was held for the first time. This is a neurological knockout tournament where teams of delegates from all WFN countries were invited to participate. Raad Shakir was the organizer of the competition, which has become extremely popular. The Australian team won it.

There were six candidates competing to organize the 18th World Congress of Neurology: Sydney (Australia), Prague (Czech Republic), Cairo (Egypt), Madrid (Spain), Bangkok (Thailand), and Tunis (Tunisia). Sydney emerged as the venue favoured by the delegates by a clear margin. Three new member countries, Bangladesh, Myanmar and United Arab Emirates, were voted WFN members, and the number of WFN members was now 89.

At the Council of Delegates, Jun Kimura was elected WFN President, and Johan A. Aarli Vice President of the WFN. Three Trustees were elected, Julien Bogousslavsky (Switzerland), William Carroll (Australia), and Roberto Sica (Argentina).

The 18th World Congress of Neurology (Sydney 2005)

President, William Carroll; Secretary-General, Geoffrey Donnan; Chairman of the Scientific Programme Committee, Sam Berkovic.

The Sydney Congress (XVIII-WCN) was held in the Sydney Convention Center on 5–11 November 2005. The congress was an outstanding success with cutting-edge neurology appropriately admixed with a broad range of topical lectures on practical neurological issues.

The Richard L. and Mary Masland Lecture was presented by Fredrik Andermann on 'Frontiers of Surgical Treatment', and the Melvyn D. Yahr lecture by Yoshikuni Mizuno on 'Progress in the Genetics of Parkinson's Disease'. As in London, the WNFo sponsored both. In addition, WNFo also presented the Eddie and Piloo Bharucha lecture for the first time, and Richard Johnson delivered it on 'Prion Diseases'. Eddie Bharucha established the first Department of Neurology in India in 1946, and served as President of the Neurological Society of India. There were also two new named lectures, which were presented at the Sydney Congress only, the John Walton Award Lecture by Salvatore DiMauro on 'Mitochondrial Neurology', funded by WNFo, and the E. Graeme Robertson Award by the recent Nobel Laureate Peter Doherty on 'Immune Memories Are Made of This'.

The Victor and Clara Soriano Award Lecture was given by Bert Sakmann, and the Fulton Society Symposium Soriano Lecture by Colin Masters on 'Therapeutic and Diagnostic Strategies Targeting A-beta Amyloid in Alzheimer's Disease'.

In addition to the regular programme, 21 countries participated in the Neurological Tournament of the Minds for a place in the finals. Six successful teams made it through to the final, and at the end the UK triumphed over Canada.

The 19th World Congress of Neurology (Bangkok 2009)

President, Niphon Poungvarin; Secretary, Somsak Laptikultham; Treasurer, Somchai Towanabut.

The 19th World Congress of Neurology took place in Bangkok, Thailand, on 24–30 October 2009 under the theme 'Innovation in Neurology'. The congress was held in the modern and unusually well-equipped conference centre Bangkok International Trade and Exhibition Centre (BITEC). The global recession had had an impact upon international travel to scientific meetings, and there had been some uncertainty about the political situation in Thailand earlier the same year, but the situation was calm and stable during the congress, which was well-organized and successful.

HRH Princess Maha Chakri Sirindhorn opened the World Congress. This was the first World Congress of Neurology with representatives from the three Chinese neurological societies, China, Taiwan, and Hong Kong.

Naraporn Prayoonwiwat chaired the Scientific Committee, together with Roger N. Rosenberg, WFN Chair of the Research Committee, and Siwaporn Chankrachang from the Education Program together with Theodore Munsat, WFN Chair of the Education Committee. Raad Shakir organized the 3rd Tournament of the Minds.

The five main themes at the congress were stroke, dementia, epilepsy, multiple sclerosis, and neuromuscular disease. Nobel Laureate Stanley Prusiner gave the Plenary Lecture on 'Biology of Prion Diseases—Lessons for other Neurodegenerative Disorders'. The Victor and Clara Soriano Award lecture was given by Vladimir Hachinski on 'Stroke: a Global Agenda', and Alastair Compston presented the Fulton Society Symposium Soriano Lecture on 'Immunogenetics and Epidemiology of Multiple Sclerosis'.

The Richard L. and Mary Masland lecture was presented by David Dodick on 'Migraine', and Roger N. Rosenberg gave the Melvin D. Yahr lecture on 'Neurodegenerative Diseases: New Strategies in Research and Therapy. Gene Vaccination for Alzheimer's Disease'. The Eddie and Pilooo Bharucha lecture was given by Thiravat Hemaducha on 'Pathophysiological Studies of Rabies in Dogs and the Role of Artificial microRNA in inhibiting Viral Replication'. A new named lecture in Bangkok was the Singhal Oration, which was given by Samuel F. Berkovic on 'Epilepsy Genetics from Basic Science to Clinical Practice'. Professor B.S. Singhal is Chair of Neurology at the Bombay Hospital Institute of Medical Sciences in Mumbai. The WNFo funded the last four named lectures.

Twenty-one countries participated in the 3rd Tournament of the Minds, which was won by the Malaysian team. There were two candidates for the office of WFN President, Vladimir Hachinski and Jagjit Chopra, and three for the position as First Vice President, Leontino Battistin, Werner Hacke and William Carroll. Vladimir Hachinski was elected President, and Werner Hacke Vice President of the WFN. Raad Shakir was the only candidate for the position as Secretary-Treasurer General.

The two WFN Medals were presented for the first time during the Bangkok congress. Noshir Wadia was awarded a medal in recognition of his service and contributions to international neurology and the WFN, and Roger Rosenberg a medal for scientific achievement on the molecular biology of Alzheimer's disease.

More than 4100 delegates from 115 countries participated, and when the Bangkok congress was over, the sum of £600,206.59 was deposited into the WFN account.

Endowed Lectures presented at the World Congresses of Neurology are The Fulton Society, Victor and Clara Soriano, and the Soriano Lectureship.

John Farquhar Fulton (1899-1960) was chair of physiology at Yale, and established the first primate physiology laboratory in the USA. One of his students was a Uruguayan neurologist, Victor Soriano, who completed a neurophysiology fellowship with Fulton. Victor and his wife Clara devoted their lives to the pursuit of neurological sciences, and established numerous symposia and also the *International Journal of Neurology*. They also founded the Fulton Society and endowed the Soriano Lectureship at the World Federation of Neurology.

The first WFN endowed lecture was made possible by a grant to the WFN from Victor and Clara Soriano. Professor Albert J. Aguayo presented The Soriano Lecture (Montreal) during the World Congress in New Delhi in 1989. The symposium during which the Soriano Lecture takes place is known as the Fulton Society Symposium.

At the Fulton Society Symposium at the World Congress of Neurology in Vancouver 1993, Professor Rita Levi-Montalcini (Rome) gave the Soriano Lecture on 'The Modulatory Role of NGF in the Nervous, Endocrine and Immune Systems'. In Buenos Aires 1997, Dr Roger N. Rosenberg (Dallas) gave the Soriano Lecture on 'The Future of Gene Therapy for Neurological Disease'. In London 2001, Dr Olle Lindvall (Lund, Sweden)'s Soriano Lecture was on

'Transplantation in Clinical Practice'. Professor Colin Masters (Melbourne) gave the Soriano Lecture at the Fulton Society Symposium in Sydney 2005 on 'Therapeutic and Diagnostic Strategies Targeting A-beta amyloid in Alzheimer's disease', in Bangkok 2009, Professor Alastair Compston (Cambridge, UK) gave the Soriano Lecture on 'Immunogenetics and Epidemiology of Multiple Sclerosis', and in Marrakesh 2011, Hidehiro Mizusawa on 'Motor Neuron'.

Thanks to a further gift from the Sorianos in 1991, the Victor and Clara Soriano Award Lecture was established at the World Congress in Vancouver in 1993. Richard T. Johnson's lecture was on 'Emerging Infections of the Nervous System'. In 1997, Stanley B. Prusiner (San Francisco) spoke about 'Prions and Neurological Disorders'. In London 2001, Francis Collins' (Bethesda, USA) topic was 'The Human Genome Project', in Sydney 2005 Bert Sakmann (Heidelberg) had chosen 'Ion Channel Physiology and Network Connectivity in the Brain, especially as relating to Epilepsy', while the topic for Vladimir Hachinski's Victor and Clara Soriano Award Lecture in Bangkok 2009 was 'Stroke: A Global Agenda'.

Support to young neurologists in training

The WFN has established scholar programmes to encourage young neurologists to undertake original work in teaching and research. Those eligible have to be under 35 years of age, and the support has mainly been related to world congresses of neurology.

Junior Travelling Fellowships are provided for young neurologists from countries classified by the World Bank as low or lower middle income to attend approved international meetings. There are 40 awards; applicants should hold a post not above that of Associate Professor and be no older than 42 years of age.

The WFN medals

Raad Shakir proposed in 2008 that the WFN should establish two WFN medals, one for service to neurology and one for achievement in neurology. The Trustees approved and decided that the first two WFN medals be presented during the World Congress of Neurology in Bangkok.

Nominations for the medals may be made either by the WFN member societies or by individual members of a member society, and have to be seconded by at least five neurologists, at least three of them from other WFN member societies.

During the World Congress of Neurology in Bangkok 2009, Professor Noshir Wadia, India, was awarded the WFN Medal for Service to International

Neurology, and Professor Roger Rosenberg, USA, the WFN Medal for Scientific Achievement in Neurology.

Noshir Wadia was awarded the WFN Medal for service to neurology. He has served his country and the WFN in many prestigious positions. In particular, he has contributed to the subject of tropical neurology, and his book *Neurological Practice: an Indian Perspective* illustrates the breadth and depth of his interest and expertise in this area. He was responsible for establishing and developing neurological services in Mumbai and setting standards for others in India to follow. Above all, he has trained and mentored over 100 neurologists who are now leaders in their field in India and abroad, which is perhaps his greatest legacy. His achievements in neurology are numerous. His publications span half a century, and include landmark papers delineating new clinical entities, published in the top international journals.

Roger Rosenberg was awarded with the WFN Medal for Scientific Achievement in Neurology. He has made significant contributions to the understanding of a number of genetically determined neurological diseases, especially the cerebellar ataxias, in which he was instrumental in demonstrating the trinucleotide repeat mutation underlying Machado–Joseph disease on 14q24.3–32.1 and in Alzheimer's disease. Not only was he able to define a potential biomarker for the dementia of Alzheimer's disease, based on the ratio of 130 kD/110 kD fragments of the APP, but his group has developed a DNA β-amyloid 42 gene vaccine, which has shown real promise and may be effective in reducing the soluble form of β-amyloid without the risk of meningoencephalitis, which accompanied earlier similar attempts. His extensive publication list attests to his activity and productivity. He is an inspirational researcher, clinician, and teacher, imbuing all those with whom he works with his infectious enthusiasm, as well as a thoughtful and considerate mentor in the many other fields of neurology in which he has been involved.

In Marrakesh in 2011, Lord Walton was awarded the WFN Medal for Service to International Neurology and Richard T. Johnson was awarded the WFN Medal for Scientific Achievement in Neurology. John Walton knows the World Federation of Neurology from the inside better than anyone else. He started the Research Group on Neuromuscular Disorders, and was the real founder and the Chairman of the Research Committee. He has been Editor-in-Chief of the *Journal of the Clinical Neurosciences*. He became First Vice President of the WFN during Masland's presidency. He also chaired the Committee on Constitution & Bye-laws. He was elected President of the World Federation of Neurology at the World Congress of Neurology in New Delhi in 1989 and he has served with grace and dignity. Walton's presidency became the most constructive modernization phase in the history of the WFN. His work in the

THE INTERNATIONAL (WORLD) CONGRESSES OF NEUROLOGY | **203**

House of Lords continues. His is a respected opinion whenever matters medical, scientific, or educational are discussed and he has served as member and chairman of several important committees and reports.

Professor Richard T. Johnson was awarded with the WFN Medal for Scientific Achievement in Neurology. In 1969 he came to the Johns Hopkins University School of Medicine as Dwight D. Eisenhower Professor of Neurology to found a new Department of Neurology with Guy McKhann. He developed a multidisciplinary laboratory group to study viruses in demyelinating diseases, malformations, neoplasms, and acute and chronic neurological diseases. Over 40 postdoctoral fellows from that laboratory continue to be active investigators in the field, and ten are now department chairpersons. In 1971, he was visiting Professor to Peru, in 1974 to Tehran, in 1976 to Germany, and in 1984 to Thailand. Between 1979 and 1991 he worked in a laboratory established in Lima to study measles during each winter. In 1988, he was appointed Director of the Department of Neurology. He has been a Visiting Professor at many universities throughout the world, is the recipient of numerous awards, and is a member of multiple honorary and professional societies. His work represents a legion of seminal studies in terms of understanding the mechanisms by which viruses infect the nervous system.

References

1 Shorvon SD, Weiss G, Avanzini G, Engel P, Meinardi H, Moshe S, Reynolds E, Wolf P. (2009) *International League Against Epilepsy 1909–2009: a centenary history.* Wiley Blackwell, Oxford.

2 Van Bogaert L. Presidential Report, *J Neurol Sci* 1966; **3**: 439–50.

3 Walton J. The Spice of Life. From Northumbria to World Neurology. Chapter 20: The World Federation of Neurology. Royal Society of Medicine Services, London 1993.

4 Seventh International Congress of Neurology: Fifth International Congress of Electroencephalography and Clinical Neurophysiology. *Brain* 1961; **84**(1): 141–3.

5 Nuwer MR, Lücking CH. Wave length and action potentials: history of the international federation of clinical neurophysiology. *Clin Neurophysiol* 2010: **61**(Suppl): 1–280.

Chapter 10

Epilogue

Vladimir Hachinski

'Continuity and change' is the motto of the current administration. The continuity is manifest in a stable administration at the London UK headquarters, scientifically and financially successful World Neurology Congresses and a balanced budget. The continuity is comfortable and desirable, but it risks conservatism and obsolescence in a rapidly changing and globalizing world, hence continuity as planned evolution has become a priority.

One change began when as Vice President I presented a white paper on holding World Neurology Congresses more often, for discussion by the delegates at an annual meeting in Glasgow in 2006. The four-year cycle of Congresses had been so successful that there was some resistance to a two-year cycle. The main arguments for moving to a quicker cycle was that it allowed us to hold Congresses where they would make the greatest difference, namely in regions where neurologists with limited resources and others interested in neurology could attend. A second argument was that if the Congresses took place every other year it would provide greater financial stability to the WFN. President John Aarli was strongly supportive from the beginning and the decision was made during his administration to move to a two-year cycle.

The first Congress held under the new policy took place in Marrakesh in 2011, fulfilling one of the main aims of the Aarli administration, to hold the first World Congress of Neurology on the African continent. The Congress motto was 'For Africa, With Africa'. It had special registration fees for participants from sub-Saharan Africa and no scholarship from that region to attend the Congress was denied. Additionally our Moroccan hosts made special arrangements for affordable housing for attendees from sub-Saharan Africa. Also, a commitment has been made that 20% of the proceeds of the Congress will be devoted to projects in Africa.

Another change was to redefine the mission of the WFN as 'fostering quality neurology and brain health worldwide'. By making brain health part of our mission, it expanded our role and implied that we would have to work with partners beyond our own specialty in order to help achieve this aim. Additionally, including brain health is in line with the definition of health by the WHO, 'a state of complete physical, mental, and social wellbeing, not merely the absence of disease or infirmity'.

'Fostering quality' implies that there should be standards by which quality is judged. These indeed have been developed and consist of:

1 Value, i.e. impact for relatively little investment in time, money or resources.

2 Viability. What is the outlook of a particular initiative beyond the initial funding? We favour investing in viable projects with growth potential.

3 Synergy. How can working together within the WFN or with other organizations enhance the initiative?

4 Evaluation. How will we know if we have succeeded? Even failure can provide profitable lessons if evaluated properly.

In line with upholding standards of quality assessments, a Committee made up of Askel Siva, (Chair, Turkey) Sarosh Katrak (India), and Charles Warlow (UK) developed criteria for endorsing meetings and Congresses, which require that they meet the standards and also that they should be for the benefit of societies, neurologists, and their patients and not for the personal profit of the organizers.

Having established quality criteria, we invited, for the first time, a grants competition to encourage projects initiated by our members. An initial competition took place in 2011 and the following projects were funded:

Prof. Masharip Atadzhanov, Bringing EMG/NCV Capacity to Zambia's University Teaching Hospital

Dr Thomas Bak, Scotland, Cognitive Clinics Worldwide

Dr Donna Bergen (USA) and Dr Raad Shakir (UK), Revision of ICD-10—Neurology Chapter and Beta Field Testing

Dr Philip Gorelick (USA), Prototype Survey of Diagnostic and Management Capabilities for Neurological Disorders: Stroke Survey

Dr Douglas Postels (USA), Pediatric Neurology Electronic Training Tool and Site

Dr Barbara Scherokman (USA), Neurological Education for Non-Neurologists in Developing Countries: A Web-Based Initiative

Prof. Ryuji Kaji (Japan), Educational Grant for Asian Neurology

Dr Mohammad Wasay (Pakistan), Neurology Training in Afghanistan: A Short Course

Prof. Jo Wilmshurst (South Africa), Children with Epilepsy in Developing Countries, and Training and Retaining Child Neurologists

The 2012 Grants Committee was enlarged to include several partners:

Peter Black, USA, World Federation of Neurosurgical Societies (WFNS)

Harry Chugani, USA, International Child Neurology Association (ICNA)

William Carroll, Australia, Multiple Sclerosis Research Australia (MSRA)

Richard Hughes, UK, European Federation of Neurological Societies (EFNS)

Pierre Magistretti, Switzerland, International Brain Research Organization (IBRO)

Solomon Moshe, USA, International League Against Epilepsy (ILAE)

Bo Norrving, Sweden, World Stroke Organization (WSO)

Bruce Sigsbee, USA, American Academy of Neurology (AAN)

Günther Dueschl, Germany, The Movement Disorder Society (MDS)

This probably will result in several jointly funded projects that also have the advantage of making the brain community aware of the initiatives and making sure that the resources are used synergistically.

The WFN has also sought to create alliances for specific purposes. On 30 March 2011, the World Brain Alliance was formed in Geneva comprising:

Alzheimer's Disease International (ADI)

European Brain Council (EBC)

International Brain Research Organization (IBRO)

International Child Neurology Association (ICNA)

International League against Epilepsy (ILAE)

World Federation of Neurorehabilitation (WFNR)

World Federation of Neurology (WFN)

World Federation of Neurosurgical Societies (WFNS)

World Psychiatry Association (WPA)

World Stroke Organization (WSO)

The World Brain Alliance was founded on three premises:

1 The brain is key to health and wellness.

2 Brain health and health begin with the mother's and the child's and their education.

3 Our brains are our future.

The Alliance participated in a high level ministerial meeting sponsored by the WHO and the Russian Federation, a UN consultation in June 2011 and the

General Assembly deliberations that adopted a non-communicable diseases political resolution on 19 September 2011.

The World Brain Alliance continues with its aim of helping to implement these resolutions, given that most brain disease falls into the category of non-communicable diseases. The World Brain Alliance also participated in the World Health Assembly in Geneva in May 2012.

The World Brain Alliance will also be part of the Age of the Brain programme being planned by the European Brain Council. The aim is to highlight the brain in Europe in 2014, the Americas in 2015, and so on, on a rotational basis. This is an ambitious goal that is being pursued.

The WFN has had a longstanding close collaboration with the WHO. Former President Johan Aarli was a major participant in two publications, *Neurology Atlas* and *Neurological Disorders, Public Health Challenge*. The current Secretary General, Raad Shakir is the Chair of the Expert Committee advising the revision of ICD-10 on neurological disorders and Donna Bergen is the Chair of the Applied Research Committee involved in the Mental Health Gap Initiative of the WHO.

In the spirit of collaboration and partnership of sub-specialty and related organizations, a Specialty Network has been organized by Vice President Werner Hacke, which had a very successful meeting at the time of the Congress in Marrakesh and probably some multidisciplinary focused congresses will ensue as a result of this initiative.

Donna Bergen and her committee have created criteria for interest groups to be associated with the WFN including formation of working groups in emerging areas such as outcomes research.

Every member of the Executive holds a portfolio. The largest and most challenging committee is that of Education, which is headed by Steven Sergay and Wolfgang Grisold, who work with successful complementarity and have developed a number of initiatives that will now be accelerated given that the priorities have been developed and the Committees and Task Forces have been enlarged.

Gustavo Roman leads the Latin American initiative that has resulted in the election of the WFN Regional Director by a democratic process, namely Marco Tulio Medina, who has as his responsibility working towards the development of a Latin American Federation of Neurological Societies. This potential Federation has also invited Canada and the American Academy of Neurology to join, in which case, it would become a Pan American Federation of Neurological Societies. Ruji Kaji leads the Asian Initiative that is very keen to foster neurology in the less developed parts of Asia. Johan Aarli has accepted the invitation to become the Chair of the Africa Initiative, with Alfred Njamnshi (Cameroon) and Girish Modi (South Africa) as Vice-Chairs.

The greatly expanded activities of the WFN required enhancement of the WFN infrastructure. The Trustees met in London UK, in February of 2012, at a professionally facilitated retreat to consider the advantages and disadvantages of a central office as compared to infrastructure support from a professional organization.

A central office has the advantage of a fixed location and the loyalty of its employees. It also allows for continuity. The disadvantages are that should one of the staff members become ill, go on maternity leave, or move on, it would create a mini crisis, because there is not the depth of staff to cover for such an eventuality. A further disadvantage is that with few people working in the same office, there is little opportunity for learning or using the advanced technologies that can be afforded by larger organizations.

The advantages of a large professional organization are that it has depth of knowledge and resources and a global reach. There is a constant learning environment and sharing of information, availability of state of the art technology and business performance standards. The disadvantages are that professional organizations tend to be more expensive, may have rapid turnover in personnel and may not provide the continuity offered by a central office and long term employees.

The Trustees agreed about the desirability of having a central London office complemented by services from a professional organization.

Although the term of this administration is for four years, deliberately all appointments were made for two years to allow the development of priorities, criteria and 'modus operandi'. Now the leadership and the membership of the Committees and Task Forces have been renewed and enlarged with a deliberate creation of Vice Chairs of Committees and Task Forces that facilitates continuity and has allowed recruitment of younger neurologists, more women and more individuals from diverse regions of the world.

The World Congress of Neurology was held in Vienna on 21–26 September 2013 on the theme 'Neurology in the Age of Globalization'. This was very apt, given the enlarging scope of WFN activities.

It is evident the changes that are taking place under this administration build on the work of all the administrations of the past half century, documented in the preceding chapters of this book. The success of the WFN stems from leading and adapting neurology in a rapidly globalizing world.

Successful continuity means continuous change.

Appendix 1

Memorandum and Articles of Association

THE COMPANIES ACTS 1985 AND 1989

MEMORANDUM AND ARTICLES OF ASSOCIATION OF WORLD FEDERATION OF NEUROLOGY

(As adopted by Special Resolution passed on 19 September 2000)

COMPANIES ACTS 1985 & 1989

COMPANY LIMITED BY GUARANTEE AND NOT HAVING A SHARE CAPITAL

MEMORANDUM OF ASSOCIATION OF WORLD FEDERATION OF NEUROLOGY

1. Name

The name of the Company is WORLD FEDERATION OF NEUROLOGY ('The Federation').

2. Registered Office

The registered office of the Federation is to be in England and Wales.

3. Objects

The objects of the Federation are to improve health worldwide by promoting education and research in neurology and the prevention and treatment of disorders of the nervous system ('the Objects').

4. Powers

The Federation has the following powers, which may be exercised only in furthering the Objects:

4.1 To organise, facilitate or promote congresses and symposia

4.2 To promote, carry out or encourage research and education and training

4.3 To promote best neurological practice standards

4.4 To promote professional interaction and dialogue

4.5 To publish or distribute information (including the official journal of The Federation) or sponsor publications

4.6 To promote or facilitate exchange arrangements or travel grants

4.7 To recognise, support, co-operate or liaise with regional groups of Member Societies and other bodies

4.8 To support, administer or set up other charities

4.9 To raise funds (but not by means of taxable trading)

4.10 To borrow money and give security for loans (but only in accordance with the restrictions imposed by the Charities Act 1993)

4.11 To acquire or hire property of any kind

4.12 To let or dispose of property of any kind (but only in accordance with the restrictions imposed by the Charities Act 1993)

4.13 To make grants or loans of money and to give guarantees

4.14 To set aside funds for special purposes or as reserves against future expenditure

4.15 To deposit or invest funds in any manner (but to invest only after obtaining advice from a financial expert and having regard to the suitability of investments and the need for diversification)

4.16 To delegate the management of investments to a financial expert, but only on terms that:

4.16.1 the investment policy is set down in writing for the financial expert by the Trustees

4.16.2 every transaction is reported promptly to the Trustees

4.16.3 the performance of the investments is reviewed regularly with the Trustees

4.16.4 the Trustees are entitled to cancel the delegation arrangement at any time

4.16.5 the investment policy and the delegation arrangement are reviewed at least once a year

4.16.6 all payments due to the financial expert are on a scale or at a level which is agreed in advance and are notified promptly to the Trustees on receipt

4.16.7 the financial expert must not do anything outside the powers of the Trustees

MEMORANDUM AND ARTICLES OF ASSOCIATION | **213**

4.17 To arrange for investments or other property of the Federation to be held in the name of a nominee (being a corporate body registered or having an established place of business in England or Wales) under the control of the Trustees or of a financial expert acting under their instructions and to pay any reasonable fee required

4.18 To insure the property of the Federation against any foreseeable risk and take out other insurance policies to protect the Federation when required

4.19 To insure the Trustees against the costs of a successful defence to a criminal prosecution brought against them as charity trustees or against personal liability incurred in respect of any act or omission which is or is alleged to be a breach of trust or breach of duty, unless the Trustee concerned knew that, or was reckless whether, the act or omission was a breach of trust or breach of duty

4.20 Subject to clause 5, to employ paid or unpaid agents, staff or advisers

4.21 To enter into contracts to provide services to or on behalf of other bodies

4.22 To establish subsidiary companies to assist or act as agents for the Federation

4.23 To act as trustee or manager of any property, endowment, bequest or gift

4.24 To act as trustee or nominee for charities in general and undertake and execute any charitable trusts which may lawfully be undertaken by the Federation and may be necessary or conducive to the Objects

4.25 To acquire, take over, assume, apply and deal with all or any of the assets and liabilities of the unincorporated charitable association called the World Federation of Neurology

4.26 To do anything else within the law which promotes or helps to promote the Objects.

5. Benefits to Members and Trustees

5.1 The property and funds of the Federation must be used only for promoting the Objects and do not belong to the members of the Federation but

5.1.1 Member Societies but not Trustees may be employed by or enter into contracts with the Federation and receive reasonable payment for goods or services supplied

5.1.2 Member Societies and Trustees may be paid interest at a reasonable rate on money lent to the Federation

5.1.3 Member Societies and Trustees may be paid a reasonable rent or hiring fee for property let or hired to the Federation

214 | THE HISTORY OF THE WORLD FEDERATION OF NEUROLOGY

5.2 A Trustee must not receive any payment of money or other material benefit (whether directly or indirectly) from the Federation except

5.2.1 as mentioned in clauses 4.19, 5.1.2 or 5.1.3

5.2.2 reimbursement of reasonable out-of-pocket expenses (including hotel and travel costs) actually incurred in running the Federation

5.2.3 an indemnity in respect of any liabilities properly incurred in running the Federation (including the costs of a successful defence to criminal proceedings)

5.2.4 payment to any company in which a Trustee has no more than a 1 per cent shareholding

5.2.5 in exceptional cases, other payments or benefits (but only with the written approval of the Commission in advance)

5.3 Whenever a Trustee has a personal interest in a matter to be discussed at a meeting of the Trustees or a committee the Trustee must:

5.3.1 declare an interest at or before discussion begins on the matter

5.3.2 withdraw from the meeting for that item unless expressly invited to remain in order to provide information

5.3.3 not be counted in the quorum for that part of the meeting

5.3.4 withdraw during the vote and have no vote on the matter

5.4 This clause may not be amended without the prior written consent of the Commission.

6. Limited Liability

The liability of Member Societies is limited.

7. Guarantee

Every Member Society promises, if the Federation is dissolved while it remains a Member Society or within 12 months afterwards, to pay up to £1 towards the costs of dissolution and the liabilities incurred by the Federation while the contributor was a Member Society.

8. Dissolution

8.1 If the Federation is dissolved the assets (if any) remaining after provision has been made for all its liabilities must be applied in one or more of the following ways:

8.1.1 by transfer to one or more other bodies established for exclusively charitable purposes within, the same as or similar to the Objects

MEMORANDUM AND ARTICLES OF ASSOCIATION | **215**

8.1.2 directly for the Objects or charitable purposes within or similar to the Objects

8.1.3 in such other manner consistent with charitable status as the Commission approve in writing in advance

8.2 A final report and statement of account must be sent to the Commission.

9. Interpretation

9.1 Words and expressions defined in the Articles have the same meanings in this Memorandum

9.2 References to an Act of Parliament are references to the Act as amended or re-enacted from time to time and to any subordinate legislation made under it.

COMPANIES ACTS 1985 & 1989

COMPANY LIMITED BY GUARANTEE AND NOT HAVING A SHARE CAPITAL

ARTICLES OF ASSOCIATION OF WORLD FEDERATION OF NEUROLOGY

1. Membership

1.1 The numbers of Member Societies with which the Federation proposes to be registered is unlimited

1.2 The Federation must maintain a register of Member Societies

1.3 From the end of the meeting at which these Articles are adopted the Member Societies shall be those national neurological societies throughout the world which on 19 September 2000 were Member Societies of the unincorporated charitable association called the World Federation of Neurology

1.4 A national neurological society of any country which is not a Member Society may become a Member Society if recommended by the Trustees and approved at a meeting of the Council of Delegates

1.5 Five or more qualified neurologists resident in a country or countries without a Member Society or Member Societies may together form a group and that group may become a Member Society if recommended by the Trustees and approved at a meeting of the Council of Delegates

1.6 A qualified neurologist resident in a country without a Member Society may apply to the Trustees to become an associate member and the Trustees shall determine his or her application

1.7 Membership of a Member Society is terminated if the Member Society:

    1.7.1 gives written notice of resignation to the Federation

    1.7.2 ceases to exist

    1.7.3 is at least one year in arrears in paying its annual dues and the Member Societies resolve at a meeting of the Council of Delegates that the membership be terminated but in such case the Member Society may apply to the Trustees for reinstatement on payment of the amount due and the Member Societies at a meeting of the Council of Delegates shall determine such application and (if approved) the terms of such reinstatement

    1.7.4 is removed from membership by resolution of the Member Societies at a meeting of the Council of Delegates on the recommendation of the Trustees on the ground that the Member Society's continued membership is harmful to the Federation (but only after notifying the Member Society in writing and considering the matter in the light of any written representations which the Member Society concerned puts forward within 42 clear days after receiving notice)

1.8 Associate membership of an associate member is terminated if the associate member:

    1.8.1 gives written notice of resignation to the Federation

    1.8.2 dies

    1.8.3 is at least one year in arrears in paying its annual dues and the Trustees resolve that the associate membership be terminated but in such case the member may apply to the Trustees for reinstatement on payment of the amount due and the Trustees shall determine such application and (if approved) the terms of such reinstatement

    1.8.4 is removed from associate membership by resolution of the Trustees on the ground that the associate member's continued membership is harmful to the Federation (but only after notifying the associate member in writing and considering the matter in the light of any written representations which the associate member concerned puts forward within 42 clear days after receiving notice)

1.9 Each Member Society shall pay the Federation annual dues being a sum for each individual member of that Member Society as agreed from time to time by the Member Societies at a meeting of the Council of Delegates

1.10 Each Member Society through its authorised delegate or secretary shall inform the Secretary-Treasurer General annually of the total of its individual membership

MEMORANDUM AND ARTICLES OF ASSOCIATION | **217**

1.11 Each associate member shall pay the Federation annual dues of the same amount as a Member Society pays for each of its individual members

1.12 A Member Society or associate member which or who is prevented by regulations in its, his or her own country from remitting the annual dues to the Federation shall deposit the annual dues in that country to be used by the Federation in the furtherance of the Objects.

2. Meetings of the Council of Delegates

2.1 The Member Societies are entitled to attend meetings of the Council of Delegates by an authorised delegate save that where there are two or more Member Societies from the same country they shall between them be represented by one authorized delegate only. Meetings of the Council of Delegates are called on at least 21 clear days notice specifying the business to be discussed

2.2 There is a quorum at a meeting of the Council of Delegates if the number of authorized delegates personally present is at least 15. The name of every authorized delegate personally present shall be notified to the Secretary-Treasurer General at the start of the meeting.

2.3 Each authorized delegate shall be an individual member of the Member Society (or of one of the Member Societies from the same country) for which he or she acts provided that a Member Society whose authorized delegate will not be present at a meeting of the Council of Delegates may appoint any member of that Member Society or the authorized delegate of another Member Society to act on its behalf as its authorized delegate at that meeting provided that no authorized delegate shall so act for more than three Member Societies at any meeting

2.4 Any authorized delegate who is appointed an Officer or Trustee shall cease to be an authorized delegate from the date he or she starts to hold office and the Member Society (or Member Societies) for whom he or she acts may appoint another authorized delegate from that date

2.5 The President or (if the President is unable or unwilling to do so) the First Vice President or (if the First Vice President is unable or unwilling to do so) an authorized delegate elected by those present and entitled to vote presides at a meeting of the Council of Delegates

2.6 Except where otherwise provided by the Act, every issue is decided by a majority of the votes cast

2.7 Except for the chair of the meeting, who has no vote other than a casting vote (unless the chair is an authorized delegate in which case he or she has a second or casting vote), every Member Society through an authorized delegate has one vote on each issue and where an authorized delegate is acting on behalf of two or more Member Societies from the same country such Member Societies through that authorized delegate shall have one vote between them on each issue

2.8 The chair may, with the consent of any meeting at which a quorum is present (and shall if so directed by the meeting), adjourn the meeting from time to time, and from place to place, but no business shall be transacted at any adjourned meeting other than the business which might have been transacted at the meeting from which the adjournment took place. Whenever a meeting is adjourned for 30 days or more notice of the adjourned meeting shall be given in the same manner as the original meeting. Save as aforesaid the Member Societies shall not be entitled to any notice of an adjournment, or of the business to be transacted at an adjourned meeting

2.9 A resolution put to the vote of the meeting shall be decided on a show of hands, unless, before or upon the declaration of the result of the show of hands, a poll is demanded by the chair or by at least five authorized delegates or by authorized delegates representing not less than one tenth of the total voting rights of all Member Societies. Unless a poll be so demanded a declaration by the chair that a resolution has been carried, or carried unanimously or by a particular majority, or lost, or not carried by a particular majority and an entry to that effect in the minute book of the Federation shall be conclusive evidence of the fact without proof of the number or proportion of the votes recorded in favour of or against that resolution. The demand for a poll may be withdrawn before the poll is taken

2.10 Subject to the provisions of Article 2.9, if a poll be demanded in manner aforesaid, it shall be taken at such time and place, and in such manner, as the chair shall direct, and the result of the poll shall be deemed to be the resolution of the meeting at which the poll was demanded. No poll shall be demanded on the election of a chair of a meeting, or on any question of adjournment. The demand of a poll shall not prevent the continuance of a meeting for the transaction of any business other than the question on which a poll has been demanded

2.11 An associate member may attend and speak but not vote at meetings of the Council of Delegates

2.12 The Federation must hold an AGM every year which all Member Societies, associate members, the Officers and the Trustees are entitled to attend

MEMORANDUM AND ARTICLES OF ASSOCIATION | **219**

2.13 At an AGM the Member Societies:

2.13.1 receive the accounts of the Federation for the previous financial year

2.13.2 receive the Trustees' report on the Federation's activities since the previous AGM

2.13.3 accept the retirement of those Officers who wish to retire or whose term of office is expiring and elect persons to those positions from the list submitted by the Nominating Committee

2.13.4 accept the retirement of those Elected Trustees who wish to retire or who are retiring by rotation and elect persons to be Trustees to fill the vacancies arising from the list submitted by the Nominating Committee

2.13.5 appoint auditors for the Federation

2.13.6 discuss and determine any issues of policy or deal with any other business put before them

2.14 Any meeting of the Council of Delegates which is not an AGM is an EGM

2.15 An EGM may be called at any time by the Trustees and must be called on the requisition of Member Societies pursuant to the provisions of the Act.

3. The Trustees

3.1 The Trustees as charity trustees have control of the Federation and its property and funds

3.2 The Trustees when complete consist of

3.2.1 the President

3.2.2 the First Vice President

3.2.3 the Secretary-Treasurer General

3.2.4 three persons elected in accordance with these Articles and

3.2.5 up to two persons co-opted in accordance with these Articles

3.3 Each person holding office as a Trustee at the date of the adoption of these Articles shall remain a Trustee until the 1st January following the first AGM after the meeting at which these Articles are adopted save that the Secretary-Treasurer General shall remain in office until 1st January following the second AGM after the meeting at which these Articles are adopted.

3.4 Every Trustee must sign a declaration of willingness to act as a charity trustee of the Federation before he or she is eligible to vote at any meeting of the Trustees

3.5 An Elected Trustee shall be elected at an AGM and shall hold office from the end of that AGM. The first three Elected Trustees shall be elected at the first AGM following the adoption of these Articles. One of the three Elected Trustees must retire at each AGM, the longest in office retiring first and the choice between any of equal service being made by drawing lots. An Elected Trustee so retiring may be reelected

3.6 A Trustee's term of office automatically terminates if he or she:

3.6.1 is disqualified under the Charities Act 1993 from acting as a charity trustee

3.6.2 is incapable, whether mentally or physically, of managing his or her own affairs

3.6.3 ceases to be an individual member of a Member Society or an associate member of the Federation (as the case may be)

3.6.4 resigns by written notice to the Trustees (but only if at least two Trustees will remain in office)

3.6.5 is removed by resolution of the Member Societies at a meeting of the Council of Delegates after the meeting has invited the views of the Trustee concerned and considered the matter in the light of any such views

3.7 The Trustees may at any time co-opt up to two persons as Co-opted Trustees who will hold office only until the next AGM but may be re-coopted

3.8 Every Trustee must be an individual member of a Member Society or an associate member of the Federation

3.9 A technical defect in the appointment of a Trustee of which the Trustees are unaware at the time does not invalidate decisions taken at a meeting.

4. Proceedings of Trustees

4.1 The Trustees must hold at least four meetings each year

4.2 A quorum at a meeting of the Trustees is three Trustees

4.3 A meeting of the Trustees may be held either in person or by suitable electronic means agreed by the Trustees in which all participants may communicate with all the other participants

4.4 The President or (if the President is unable or unwilling to do so) some other Trustee chosen by the Trustees present presides at each meeting

4.5 Every issue may be determined by a simple majority of the votes cast at a meeting but a written resolution signed by all the Trustees is as valid as a resolution passed at a meeting (and for this purpose the resolution may be contained in more than one document and will be treated as passed on the date of the last signature)

4.6 Except for the chair of the meeting, who has a second or casting vote, every Trustee has one vote on each issue

4.7 A procedural defect of which the Trustees are unaware at the time does not invalidate decisions taken at a meeting.

5. Powers of Trustees

The Trustees have the following powers in the administration of the Federation:

5.1 to exercise any powers of the Federation which are not reserved to a meeting of the Council of Delegates

5.2 to appoint three or more individuals, each of whom shall be an individual member of a Member Society or an associate member of the Federation, shall come from a different country and shall not be a Trustee, to form a Nominating Committee whose functions are as set out in Article 6 and whose proceedings shall not be reported to the Trustees

5.3 subject to Article 5.2, to delegate any of their functions to committees to include a Finance Committee, and these committees shall consist of three or more individuals, each of whom shall be an individual member of a Member Society or an associate member of the Federation, appointed by the Trustees and at least one of them shall be a Trustee. All proceedings of these committees must be reported promptly to the Trustees

5.4 to make Rules consistent with the Memorandum, these Articles and the Act to govern proceedings at meetings of the Council of Delegates

5.5 to make Rules consistent with the Memorandum, these Articles and the Act to govern proceedings at their meetings and at meetings of committees

5.6 to make Rules consistent with the Memorandum, these Articles and the Act to govern the administration of the Federation and the use of its seal (if any)

5.7 to establish procedures to assist the resolution of disputes within the Federation.

6. Nominating Committee

The functions of the Nominating Committee are:

6.1 to choose a list of candidates for the offices of Trustee and Officer other than Additional Officer

6.2 to publish that list at least six months prior to the relevant AGM

6.3 to accept additional nominations supported with the signatures of five or more authorized delegates which are received by the Secretary- Treasurer General at least thirty days prior to that AGM

6.4 to submit the amended list at that AGM.

7. Officers

7.1 The Officers of the Federation shall be the President, the first Vice President, the Secretary-Treasurer General and such other Vice Presidents as the Member Societies at a meeting of the Council of Delegates shall decide and such Additional Officers as the Trustees shall decide

7.2 The Officers shall be elected at an AGM and shall hold office from 1st January following that AGM until 1st January following the fourth AGM after that AGM and only the Secretary-Treasurer General may be re-appointed and then only for one further term of office

7.3 The Secretary-Treasurer General will act as the Secretary of the Federation in accordance with the Act

7.4 If an Officer does not complete his or her term of office the Trustees may fill that vacancy for the unexpired term except that if the office of President becomes vacant the first Vice President shall assume the responsibilities of the President until the next AGM when a new President shall be elected to hold office for the unexpired term then remaining of the previous President and at the expiration of that term may be re-elected but only for one further term of office

7.5 Every Officer must be an individual member of a Member Society or an associate member of the Federation

7.6 The Trustees may appoint as an Additional Officer of the Federation any individual member of a Member Society or an associate member of the Federation upon such terms and with such title as the Trustees shall decide.

8. Records & Accounts

8.1 The Trustees must comply with the requirements of the Act and of the Charities Act 1993 as to keeping financial records, the audit of accounts and the preparation and transmission to the Registrar of Companies and the Commission of:

8.1.1 annual reports

8.1.2 annual returns

8.1.3 annual statements of account

8.2 The Trustees must keep proper records of

8.2.1 all proceedings at general meetings of the Council of Delegates

8.2.2 all proceedings at meetings of the Trustees

8.2.3 all reports of committees and

8.2.4 all professional advice obtained

8.3 Accounting records relating to the Federation must be made available for inspection by any Trustee at any reasonable time during normal office hours and may be made available for inspection by Member Societies if the Trustees so decide

8.4 A copy of the Federation's latest available statement of account must be supplied on request to any Trustee or Member Society, or to any other person who makes a written request and pays the Federation's reasonable costs, within two months.

9. Notices

9.1 Notices under these Articles may be sent by hand, or by post or by suitable electronic means or (where applicable to Member Societies generally) may be published in any suitable journal or any newsletter distributed by the Federation

9.2 The only address at which a Member Society is entitled to receive notices is the address shown in the register of Member Societies

9.3 Any notice given in accordance with these Articles is to be treated for all purposes as having been received

9.3.1 48 hours after being sent by electronic means or delivered by hand to the relevant address

9.3.2 two clear days after being sent by first class post to that address

9.3.3 ten clear days after being sent by overseas post to that address

9.3.4 on being handed to the authorized delegate of a Member Society personally or, if earlier,

9.3.5 as soon as the Member Society acknowledges actual receipt

9.4 A technical defect in the giving of notice of which the Trustees are unaware at the time does not invalidate decisions taken at a meeting.

10. Dissolution

The provisions of the Memorandum relating to dissolution of the Federation take effect as though repeated here.

11. Interpretation

11.1 In the Memorandum and in these Articles:

'The Act' means the Companies Act 1985

'Additional Officer' means an Officer of the Federation appointed pursuant to Article 7.6

'AGM' means an annual general meeting of the Federation

'these Articles' means these articles of association

'authorized delegate' means an individual who is authorized by a Member Society (or Member Societies from the same country) to act on its (or their) behalf at meetings of the Council of Delegates and whose name is given to the Secretary by the Member Society (or Member Societies)

'the Federation' means the company governed by these Articles

'charity trustee' has the meaning prescribed by section 97(1) of the Charities Act 1993

'clear day' means 24 hours from midnight following the relevant event

'the Commission' means the Charity Commissioners for England and Wales

'Co-opted Trustees' means the persons referred to in Article 3.2.5

'country' means a country as determined by the Trustees

'EGM' means an extraordinary general meeting of the Federation

'Elected Trustees' means the persons referred to in Article 3.2.4

'financial expert' means an individual, company or firm who is an authorized person or an exempted person within the meaning of the Financial Services Act 1986

'First Vice President' means the First Vice President of the Federation

'meeting of the Council of Delegates' means a general meeting of the Federation

'material benefit' means a benefit which may not be financial but has a monetary value

'Member Society' and 'Member Societies' mean respectively a member and members of the Federation 'membership' where the context so admits refers to membership of the Federation

'Memorandum' means the Federation's Memorandum of Association

'the Objects' means the Objects of the Federation as defined in clause 3 of the Memorandum

'Secretary-Treasurer General' means the Secretary-Treasurer General of the Federation

'President' means the President of the Federation

'taxable trading' means carrying on a trade or business on a continuing basis for the principal purpose of raising funds and not for the purpose of actually carrying out the Objects

'Trustee' means a director of the Federation and 'Trustees' means all of the directors

'written' or 'in writing' refers to a legible document on paper including a fax message

'year' means calendar year

11.2 Expressions defined in the Act have the same meaning

11.3 References to an Act of Parliament are to the Act as amended or re-enacted from time to time and to any subordinate legislation made under it.

Index

Page numbers in *italics* indicate photographs.

A

Aarli, J.A. 69, 73–5, *74*, 76, *77*, 77–9, 98, 99, 104, 144, 148, 167, 170, 171–2, 198, 205, 208
Abada, M. 162
Acheson, E.D. 117
Acta Neuropathologica 24, 55, 104, 122, 124, 144–5
Ad-hoc Strategic Planning Group Meeting, Sopwell House (1999) 66
Adams, R. 97
Adeloye, A. 162
Administrator of the Federation 63
Africa 42, 76
Africa Committee 76
Africa Initiative 75, 163–4, 208
Agnoli, A. 134
Aguayo, A.J. 195, 200
Al Deeb, S. 69
Alajouanine, T. 7, 8, 190
Alema, G. 189
Allen, A.R. 2
Altman, R. 28
Amaducci, L. 127, 128
Amayo, E. 76
American Academy of Neurology 12, 15, 150
Amyotrophic Lateral Sclerosis and Related Motor Neuron Disorders 130
Andermann, E. 123
Andermann, F. 198
André–Thomas 7, 8, 190
annual dues 21, 32, 48, 94–5, 113
Annual General Meetings 72, 88
Appel, L. 125
Applied Research Committee 109
Arana-Iñiguez, R. 16, 31, 157
Arezki, M. 76
Arizaga, R. 128
Articles of Association 71–2, 90, 211–25
Asbury, A. 58, 97
Asenjo, A. 7, 16, 158
Asia Initiative 156–7
Asian Oceanian Association of Neurology (AOAN) 150, 151–3
Atadzhanov, M. 206
Australian Association of Neurologists 155–6

B

Babinski, J. 2, 9
Bailey, P. 11, 12, 14–16, 17, *21*, 27, 30, 31, 32, 38, 86, 87, 90–1, 95, 139, 150, 159, 173–4, 190
Bak, T.H. 120, 206
Baker, A.B. 12, 26
Barac, B. 133
Barbeau, A. 41, 47, 126
Barcia Goyanes, J.J. 16
Barlow, T. 1
Barnes, M. 132
Barnett, H.J. 98, 195, 196
Barraquer Bordas, I. 192
Barrows, Professor 101
Bartko, D. 165
Batten, F. 2
Battistin, L. 69, 99
Bauer, H. 117, *118*, 194
Bay, E. 97, 119
Becker, C. 106
Behavioral Neurology International 136
Belloni, G. 16, *16*, *21*
Ben-Hamida, M. 162, 164
Bender, M.B. 191
Benton, A. 119
Bergen, D. 115, 206, 208
Berkovic, S. 156, 198, 200
Berman, S. 16, 160–1
Bertolote, J. 76
Bharucha, E.P. 17, 30, 31, 97, 194, 198
Bick, K. 127
Bilger, S. 72
Bill, P. 76, 162
Bini, L. 6
Birbeck, G.L. 103
Black, P. 207
Blessed, G. 127
Bodechtel, G. 190
Bogousslavsky, J. 50, 69, 73, 74, 99, 198
Bojinov, S. 16, *16*
Bolis, D. 50
Borg, J. 132
Born–Bunge Foundation 18
Bornstein, N.M. 141
Boukhrissi, N. 162
Bradley, W. 171
Brante, G. 117, *118*
Bruyn, G. 48, 51, 54, 92, 93–4, 97, 113, 140, 192

Bunge, E. 18
Bunge Institute 18, 19, 33

C

Calne, D. 133, 197
Canadian Neurological Sciences Federation 150
Carroll, W. 69, 99, 156, 198, 207
Castaigne, P. 26
Castell-Diaz, C. 17
Caxias 176–9, 181–2
Cerebrovascular Disease Project (CVDP) 25–7
Cernacek, J. 97
Cervos-Navarro 135
Chana, P. 69
Chandy, J. 173
Chankrachang, S. 199
Charcot Award 131
Charities Aid Foundation consultation 60–2, 63
charity status 62
Cheung, R. 77
Chi, L. 79
Chinese Neurological Society 77–9
Chitanwudth, H. 25, 126
Chopra, J.S. 57, 98, 99, 133, 143, 194
Chouza, C. 69
Christiansen, V. 6
Chugani, H. 207
Clarke, R.H. 2
Coërs, C. 24, 121
collaboration 41
Collins, F. 198, 201
Collomb, H. 162
Committee for the Decentralization Plan 30
committees of WFN 89–90
Compston, A. 199, 201
Constitution & Bye-Laws Committee 70
Continuing Education Committee 100–3
Continuum: Lifelong Learning in Neurology
programme 67, 102, 145
corporate status 61, 67–8, 70–1
Council of Delegates 39, 67, 87–8, 89, 99
Couto, D. 17, 158, 159
Cox, L.B. 155
Critchley, M. 5, 11, 12, *16*, 17, *21*, 25, 29, 33,
34–7, *34*, 38, 39, 41, 42, 86, 87, 95, 97, 119,
139, 190, 191
Cruz-Sanchez, F. 124
Csanda, E. 51
Culebras, A. 50, 98, 105, 106, 107, 134
Cummings, J.L. 117, *118*
*Current Opinions in Neurology and
Neurosurgery* 101
Currier, R.D. 126

D

Dada, O. 162, 193
Daroff, R. 54, 62, 72, 94, 103, 142, 196

De Rojas, C. 17, *21*
Decade of the Brain 63–4
Decentralization Plan 30–1, 86–7, 150–2
Dejerine, J.J. 2, 7
DeJong, R.N. 17, 30
Del Brutto, O. 126
demyelinating disease 9
Den Hartog Jager, A.A. 192
DiMauro, S. 198
Dipp, M.T. 152
Divry, P. 8
Dodick, D. 199
Doherty, P. 198
Donaghy, M. 90, 99
Donnan, G. 156, 198
Dore-Duffy, P. 140
Doussou, G.A. 152
Dreyfus, P. 50, 52, 92
Du Pré Grants 131
Dua, T. 75, 171
dues 21, 32, 48, 94–5, 113
Dueschl, G. 207
Dumas, M. 76, 162
Durr, A. 127

E

E. Graeme Robertson Award Lecture 198
ECT 6
Eddie and Piloo Bharucha Lecture 198, 199
Edgar, G. 117, *118*
education 56, 67, 100–3, 145, 208
Education Committee 102, 103
Education of Non-neurologists in Developing
Countries 103
Ehrlich, P. 2
El-Benhawy, A. 164
El-Deeb, S. 164
El-Gindi, S. 162
El-Kurdi, A. 164
El-Tamawy, M.S 76
Elected Trustees 89, 99
electroconvulsive therapy 6
electroencephalograph 5, 7
Endowed Lectureships 105, 195, 197, 198,
200–1
Engel, J. 145
Engel, P. 102
Engel, W.K. 15
epilepsy 2–3, 5, 8
Epilepsy International 56
EspadalerMedina, J. 17, 93, 192
Etribi, A. 164
European Federation of Neurological Societies
(EFNS) 59, 150, 164–6
European Neurological Society 166
Executive Committee
meetings 32–3, 38, 40, 159–60
power of 86–7

F

Fadli, E. 164
Fahn, S. 197
Fankhauser, R. 115, 124
Fazekas, F. 141
Fazio, C. 134
Feldman, S. 53, 194
Finance Committee 48, 54–5, 93–4
financial issues 21–2, 26, 31–3, 40, 46, 47–8,
      53–5, 90–6, 113
Finkel, M. 107
Fischgold, H. 25, 125
Flores, A. 8, 190
Fog, T. 131
Folch-Pi, J. 117, *118*
Franceschetti, A. 24, 33–4, 38, 39, 110, 111–12,
      115, 123
Frauchiger, E. 17, 24, 38, 39, 112, 115
Freeman, R. 127
Freeman, W. 5
Friedrichs, M. 141
Fulton, J.F. 5, 200
Fulton Society Symposium Soriano
      Lecture 195, 196, 198, 199, 200–1
Fund-Raising Subcommittee 54

G

Gajdusek, D.C. 15
Gallo Diop, A. 76, 196
Game, J. 97
Gänshirt, H. 194
Garcin, R. 7, 9, 17, 24, 31, 121, 159, 190
Gastaut, H. 8
Geoffroy, G. 28
Gerstenbrand, F. 98, 125, 131, 134, 165
Gibbs, C.J. 15
Giordano, C. 162
Glaser, G.H. 23, 28, 122, 139
Godwin-Austen, R. 57, 63, 64, 69, 72, 73, 74,
      106, 197
Gold, L. 196
Gorelick, P. 206
Gotoh, L.F. 134
Gouider, R. 152, 164
Gozzano, M. 189
Gracevic, N. 135
Grants Committee 206–7
Grashchenkov, N. 17, 28
Griggs, R. 152
Grisold, W. 208
Guevara, M. 158
Guillain, G.C. 8, 190

H

Hachinski, V. 72, 73, 99, 156–7, 196, 199, 200,
      201
Hacke, W. 99, 196, 200, 208
Haimanot, R.T. 76, 162

Hallett, M. 143–4
Halmagyi, G.M. 124
Halpern, L. 17
Hamida, B. 58, 97
Hanley, D. 130
Harding, A. 123, 126, 166
Hashem, S. 164
Hausmanowa-Petrusewicz, I. 24, 53,
      121, 194
Heijstee, A.P.J. 192
Heiss, W.-D. 99
Hemaducha, T. 199
Henner, K. 17, 25, 132
Herman, E. *16*, 17, 97
Herskovits, E. 53, 194
Hicham, C. 76
Hoff, H. 30, 190
Hokkanen, E. 98, 184
Holmes, G. 4, 5, 6, 8, 190
Hommes, O.R. 141
Honduras training programme 103
Hong Kong Neurological Society 79
Horsley, V. 2, 9
Horsley–Clarke frame 2
Hughes, R. 152, 197, 207
Hutton, S.E. 140
Hyllested, K. 23, 117

I

Income from World Congresses 95–6
International Bureau for Epilepsy 3
International Child Neurology
      Association 122
International Classification of Diseases
      (ICD) 56, 171
International Congress of Neuroimmunology
      (1982) 56
International Congress of Neurology
      1931 Berne 3–4
      1935 London 4–5
      1939 Copenhagen 6
      1949 Paris 7
      1953 Lisbon 7–8
      1957 Brussels 8–10
International Congress of Psychiatry,
      Neurology, Psychology and Care of the
      Insane (Amsterdam 1907) 2–3
International EEG Congress 7
International Federation of Clinical
      Neurophysiology 64
International Federation of Multiple Sclerosis
      Societies 131
International Federation of Societies for EEG
      and Clinical Neurophysiology
      (IFSECN) 136
International League Against Epilepsy
      (ILAE) 2–3, 5, 6, 8, 55–6, 135, 187
International Pediatric MS Study Group 131

International Society for Paediatric
   Neurology 122
International Society of
   Neuroimmunology 135
International Society of Neurovirology 135
International Stroke Society (ISS) 50

J

Jackson, J.H. 5
Jacobsen, C. 5
Janeway, R. 106
Japanese Society for Neurochemistry 119
Japanese Society of Neurology 154–5
Jefferson, G. 9
John Walton Award Lecture 198
Johnson, R. 135, 195, 198, 201, 202, 203
Journal de Génétique Humaine 123
Journal of Neuroimmunology 104, 135
Journal of the Neurological Sciences 22, 28–9,
   47, 51, 55, 104, 139–41
Jung, R. 194
Junior Travelling Fellowships 201
Juul-Jensen, P. 45, 48, 50, 92, 93, 95, 192

K

Kaji, R. 99, 154, 206, 208
Kalaria, R. 76
Kaps, M. 133
Katabira, E. 76
Katrak, S. 206
Katsuki, S. 51, 155, 193
Katzman, R. 56
Kety, S. 15
Khalifa, A. 152, 164
Khalili, K. 135
Kieseier, B.C. 141
Kim, J.S. 69
Kimura, J. 57–8, 62, 64, 67, *68*, 68–71,
   73, 77, 90, 98, 154, 170, 183–5, 196,
   197, 198
Kinnier Wilson, S.A. 4–5
Klein, D. 23, 33–4, 39, 49, 93, 110, 111, 113,
   115, 123, 126, 134
Klimkova-Deutschova, E. 129
Korczyn, A. 105, 127, 141
Korey, S. 117, *118*
Kornyev, S. 17
Kouassi, B. 76
Krabbe, K. 6, 8, 17, 190
Kreindler, A. 17
Kroll, M.B. 4
Kugelberg, E. 17
Kurdi, A. 152
Kure, S. 154
Kurland, L. 23, 28, 117
Kurtzke, J. 23, 117
Kuzuhara, S. 154

L

Lance, J.W. 58, 98
Laptikultham, S. 199
Latin American Federation of Neurological
   Societies 208
Lea-Plaza, H. 159
Lechner, H. 49, 54, 134, 135
Lennox, W.G. 5
Leonhard, K. 191
Lesney, I. 122
Levi-Montalcini, R. 195, 200
Lewis, R.A. 140
Lhermitte, F. 26
Liaison Committees 29
Liberson, W.T. 7
Lima, P.A. 5, 8, 178
Lindvall, O. 198, 200
Lisak, R.P. 140
Liu, C.-K. 79
lobotomy 5
Loeb, C. 49, 51, 134, 135
Long Range Planning Committee 89
Lopez-Ibor, J. 17
Lowenthal, A. 11, 23, 28, 53, 56, 98, 113, 115,
   117, *118*, 136, 139, 141, 159, 196
Lu, C.-Z. 77, *77*, 78, 79
Ludolph, A. 131
Lukas, E. 129

M

MacCarthy, C.S. 191
MacDonald, I. 197
Macdonald Critchley Lecture 197
McDonald Fellowship 131
McLeod, J.G. 97
McNaughton, F. 97
Maffei, W.E. 25, 126
Magistretti, P. 207
Manes, F. 120
Mannen, T. 184
Marburg, O. 3, *3*
Marin, O. 174
Marsden Memorial Lecture 197
Marshall, J. 49, 134, 135
Martinez-Lage, J.M. 53, 194
Masdeu, J.C. 125
Masland, R.L. 50–3, *51*, 55–6, 57, 97, 142,
   161, 170
Masters, C. 199, 201
Matthews, B. 140
Matthews, W.B. 47, 51
Matzke, H.A. 23, 121
medals 200, 201–3
Medina, M. 103, 208
Mehndiratta, M.M. 153
Melvin D. Yahr lecture 105, 197,
   198, 199
Membership Committee 103

INDEX | **231**

Memorandum and Articles of Association
71–2, 90, 211–25
Menken, M. 101
mental health 169–70
mental health Gap Action Programme 171
Merritt, H. 9, 11–12, 13–14, 17, *21*, 26, 31, 86,
150, 159, 173, 189, 190, 191
Mertens, H.-G. 194
Mesulam, M. 120
Meyer, J.S. 49, 134, 135
mhGAP Forum 171
Miladi, N. 69
Miller, H. 39, 40, 41, *42*, 42–4, 91, 93, 191
Minager, A. 141
Miura, K. 154
Mizuno, Y. 198
Mizusawa, H. 201
modernization of WFN governance 61–3
Modi, G. 76, 208
Moniz, E. 5, 8
Monrad-Krohn, G.H. 8, 9, 17, 190
Moossy, J. 26
Moshe, S. 207
Mottura, G. 26
Muchnik, S. 196
Mülle, D. 191
multiple sclerosis 9
Munsat, T. 63, 67, 69, 72, 97, 99, 102, *102*,
115, 145, 199
Murray, J. 101, 105
Mustafa, M. 51

N

Nachev, S. 17
Narabayashi, H. 53, 194
National Institute of Neurological Diseases and
Blindness (NINDB) 12, 15
Ndiaye, I.P. 162
*Neurological Disorders: Public Health
Challenges* 170–1
neurological education 56, 67, 100–3,
145, 208
Neurological Society of India 153–4
Neurological Tournament of the Mind 198,
199, 200
Neurology 12, 15
Neurology Atlas 170
Neuromuscular Disorders 121
neurosurgery 6, 7, 9
Newell, F.W. 24, 123
newsletter of WFN (*World Neurology*) 53, 57,
104, 141–4, 194
Newton, K. 63, 70, 72, 73, 76, 90, 106
Njamnshi, A. 76, 152, 208
Nominating Committee 96–7, 98, 99–100
Norrving, B. 207
North American Association of
Neurology 150

O

Obrda, Dr 24, 132
Okinaka, S. 17, 31, 152
Olesen, J. 166, 197
Olivarius, B. de Fine 45, 47–8, 91–2, 97, 192
O'Malley, C.D. 24
Oppenheim, H. 2
Orgogozo, J.-M. 171
Osuntokun, B.O. 126

P

Pan African Association of Neurological
Sciences (PAANS) *42*, 150, 160–2
Pan American Association of Neurology 150,
157–8
Pan American Congress of Neurology 87,
158–60
Pan American Federation of Neurological
Societies 208
Pan Arab Union of Neurological Societies
(PAUNS) 150, 164
Pan European Society of Neurology 165
Parkinsonism 9, 47
Parkinsonism and Related Disorders 133–4
Paty, D. 98, 104, 171, 195
Pavlov, I. 5
Pearse, E. 117, *118*
Pedley, T. 197
Penfield, W. 5, 159
Pereyra-Käfer, J. 17, 157
phenytoin 13
Pinelli, P. 98, 196
Poch, G. 158
Poech, G. 97
Poeck, K. 58, 93, 97, 98, 101, 115, 194, 196
Policy Committee 17, 32, 88
Pool, J.L. 191
Portera-Sanchez, A. 58, 97
Poser, C. 11, 12, *21*, 26, 27, *27*, 117, *118*, 139,
150, 151, 152, 154, 155, 174
Postels, D. 206
Poungvarin, N. 199
Prayoonwiwat, N. 199
prions 15
Problem Commissions 22–3, 32, 39, 110,
112–13, 116, 188
Cerebral Palsy 24
Comparative Neuroanatomy 23, 121
Developmental Neurology 23, 122
EEG-Neurophysiology 25
Geographical Neurology, Statistics and
Epidemiology 23, 116–17
History of Neurology 24, 119
Language Disorders (Aphasiology) 119–20
Neuro-anaesthesia 23
Neurochemistry 23, 117–19
Neurogenetics 23, 123
Neurological Rehabilitation 25

Problem Commissions (*continued*)
Neuromuscular Diseases 24, 121
Neuro-oncology 24, 122
Neuro-ophthalmology and Neuro-
otology 24, 123
Neuropathology, Comparative
Neuropathology and Neuro-
oncology 24, 124
Neuroradiology 24–5, 125
Rehabilitation and Physical Medicine
131–2
Tropical Neurology 25, 126
Prockop, L. 129
professional management 73, 209
Project Atlas 170
Prusiner, S. 195, 199, 201
Pruzanski, W. 28
Public Relations Committee 104, 171–2
Publications Subcommittee 54, 103–4

Q

qualified neurologists 147–8
quality assessment 205–6
Quandt, J. 191
Quastel, J. 117, *118*

R

Ramamurthi, B. 17, *21*, 173
Rascol, A. 98, 196
Refsum, S. 17, 26, 28, 44–7, *45*, 48, 50, 95, 97,
192, 193
Regional Directors 168
Regional Vice Presidents 167–8
regions of WFN 148–50, 167, 168
Research Advances in Neurology
(website) 115
Research and Continuing Education
Committee 67
Research Committee 39–40, 47, 48–50, 109,
110, 111, 114–15
chairs 115
guidelines for Research Groups 136–7
neurological education 101–3
Research Groups 37–8, 39–40, 41, 47, 55, 109,
112–13
Aging and Dementia 56
Aphasia/Cognitive Disorders 119–20
Ataxia 126–7
Autonomic Disorders 127
Behavioural Neurology 56
Cerebral Circulation 134
Cerebrospinal Fluid 136
Cerebrovascular Disease 49–50, 134–5
Clinical Neuropharmacology 127
Comparative Neuroanatomy 121
Delivery of Neurological Services 101
Dementia 127–9
Environmental Neurology 129

Extrapyramidal Disorders 116, 133–4
guidelines 136–7
Huntington's Disease 130
Intensive Care Neurology 130
Migraine and Headache 130
Motor Neuron Diseases 130–1
Multiple Sclerosis 131
Neuro-anaesthesiology 122
Neuroethics 131
Neurogenetics 123
Neuroimaging 125
Neuroimmunology and Neurovirology 56,
135
Neurological Education (later Medical
Education) 100–1
Neuromuscular Diseases 121
Neuro-oncology 122
Neuro-ophthalmology and Neuro-
otology 124
Neuropaediatrics 122
Neuropathology 124
Neuroradiology 125
Neuro-rehabilitation and Restorative
Neurology 131–2
Neurosonology (previously Ultrasonics in
Neurology) 132–3
Neurotoxicology 129–30
Neurotraumatology 135–6
Organization and Delivery of Care 133
Palliative Care 133
Parkinsonism and Related Disorders
133–4
Sleep 134
Space and Underwater Neurology 134
Reuck, J. de 152
Ribière, G. 23, 120, 122
Richard L and Mary Masland Lecture 105,
197, 198, 199
Richter, D. 117, *118*
Riley, H.A. 3, 8, 190
Robertson, E.G. 30, 97, 139, 155–6
Robinson, R.G. 31
Robles de Hernandez, A.M. 152
Roizin, L. 129
Roman, G. 208
Roos, R. 130
Rose, F.C. 57, 58, 97, 98, 142–3, 195,
196, 197
Rosenberg, R. 69, 72, 99, 102, 115, 196, 199,
200, 202
Rosser, M. 197
Roth, M. 127
Rothmann, M. 2
Rowland, L.P. 13–16
Ruberti, R. 42, 161, 162
RubioDonnadieu, F. 98, 158, 160
Russell, D. 179
Rutishauser, E. 26

S

Sachs, B. 3, *3*, 4, 6
Sachs, E. 9
Sahs, A.L. 159
Said, G. 121, 166
Sakmann, B. 199, 201
Salzburg Conference on Cerebral Vascular Disease 49–50
San Luis, A. 152
Sánchez-Longo, L.P. 160
Sanvito, W.L. 125
Saraceno, B. 75, 171
Sarkisov, S.A. 17
Sartorius, N. 56, 64, 170
Satoyoshi, E. 57–8, 97, 98, 155, 184, 196
Saxena, S. 75, 171
Schaltenbrand, G. *16*, 17, 86, 97, 119
Scherokman, B. 206
scholars programmes 201
Schultze, Dr 193
Secretariat, making permanent 63
Secretary-Treasurer General 90–1, 99
Seitelberger, F. 24, 124, 144, 190
Seminars in Clinical Neurology 102, 145
Sepich, M. 159
Sercl, M. 17
Sergay, S. 208
Shakir, R. 74, 76, 78, 99, 171, 198, 199, 200, 201, 208
Sherrington, C. 3, 5, 6, 9
Shibasaki, H. 185
Shy, G.M. 15
Sica, R. 69, 98, 99, 196, 198
Sierra, A.M. 4
Sigsbee, B. 207
Silberberg, D. 100
Silberstein, S.D. 130
Sillevis-Smitt, C. 17
Singhal, B.S. 101, 152, 200
Singhal Oration 200
Siva, A. 206
Soriano Lecture 195, 196, 198, 199, 200–1
Sorour, O. 161
Specialty Network 208
Spiller, W.G. 2
Spina-Franca, A. 51, 97
Steering Committee 17, 55, 88–9
Stein, R. 76
Stephan, H. 23, 121
Stramignoni, Dr. 26
Stroke 135
Stroke Affairs Committee 135
stroke organizations 50
Subirana, A. 192
Sükrü Aksel, I. *16*, 17
Svennerholm, L. 117, *118*
Swash, M. 130
Swift, T.R. 152

T

Taiwanese Neurological Society 77, 79
Tamraz, J. 125
Task and Advisory Force for Neurology in Africa (TAFNA) 76
Tcheazi, E *21*
Tchehrazi, E. 17
teleconferences 145
Terry, B. 159
Terry, H.R. 23
Thage, O. 93
Thiébaut, F. 17, 31
Thieffry, S. 23, 122
Third World Medical Research Foundation 114
Thomas, P.K. 166
Tomlinson, B. 56, 127
Toole, J.F. 50, 52, 53, 56, 57, 64–7, *65*, 92, 98, 104–5, 106, 140, 142, 145, 170, 195, 196, 197
Toselli, L.B. 196
Tournay, A. 2, 11, 17, 86
Tourtellotte, W. 117, *118*
Towanabut, S. 199
Toyokura, Y. 155
training 76, 103
Trelles, O.M. 17, *21*, 87, 139, 157–8, 159, 160, 174
Trojaborg, W. 24, 121
Trustees 89, 99
Tsai, C.-P. *77*, 79, 153
Tschabitscher, H. 96, 165, 190
Tsubaki, T. 155, 193

U

Usunov, G, *16*

V

Valasco-Suarez 97
van Bogaert, A. 19
van Bogaert, L. 6, 8, 11, 12, 17–22, *18*, *21*, 26, 27, 28, 30, 31, 32–3, 38, 39, 85–6, 87, 93, 110, 117, *118*, 126, 139, 150, 151, 157, 158, 159, 173, 174, 187, 188, 190, 191
van der Lugt, L.P.M. 100
van Gehuchten, P. 8, 190
Vecsei, L. 141
Vernon, D.C. 67, 105, 106
Victor and Clara Soriano Award Lecture 198, 199, 200, 201
Visser, M. de 69, 72, 99
Voltz, R. 133
Vourc'h, G. 23

W

Wadia, N. 25, 58, 98, 126, 147, 173–83, *180*, *182*, 200, 201–2
Walker, E. 191
Walker, S. 56

Walshe, F. 8, 9
Walton, J. 24, 28, 29, 39, 41, 47, 48, 50, 53, 55,
    56, 57, *58*, 58–60, 77, 93, 97, 98, 110, 111,
    113, 114, 115, 120, 121, 123, 139, 140, 155,
    171, 185, 195, 196, 202–3
Walton, S. 136
Warlow, C. 197, 206
Wasay, M. 206
websites 115, 144
Wender, M. 165
Whitehouse, P. 127
WHO Liaison Committee 104
Wilmshurst, J. 206
Winther, K. 17
Wohlfart, G. *16*, 17
Wolters, E. 134
World Association of Neurological
    Commissions (WANC) 33–4, 38–9,
    40, 110
World Brain Alliance 207–8
World Congress of Medicine (London
    1913) 1–2
World Congress of Neurology/Neurlological
    Sciences
    1957 Brussels 8–10, 187
    1961 Rome 31, 189–90
    1965 Vienna 190–1
    1969 New York 191–2
    1973 Barcelona 192
    1977 Amsterdam 192–3
    1981 Kyoto 193–4
    1985 Hamburg 194
    1989 New Delhi 194–5
    1993 Vancouver 195–6
    1997 Buenos Aires 196–7

2001 London 197–8
2005 Sydney 198–9
2009 Bangkok 199–200
2011 Marrakesh 156, 202, 205
2013 Vienna 209
World Federation for Neuro-
    rehabilitation 132
World Health Organization (WHO) 41, 50,
    56, 64, 68, 75, 148, 149–50, 167, 168–9,
    170–1, 208
World Muscle Society 121
World Neurology (journal) 22, 27–8, 55, 57–8,
    139, 155
World Neurology (newsletter of WFN) 53, 57,
    104, 141–4, 194
World Neurology Foundation 104–7
World Neurology Research and Education
    Foundation 105
World Sleep Day 134
World Stroke Federation (WSF) 50
World Stroke Organization 50

Y
Yahr, M. 38, 47, 116, 133, 191, 197–8
Yates, P.O. 26
Yatsu, F. 184
York, G. 119

Z
Zec, N. 17
Zenebe, M. 76
Zhi, L. 79
Zivadinov, R. 141
Zou, H. 79
Zülch, K. 24, 38, 49, 122, 134, 194